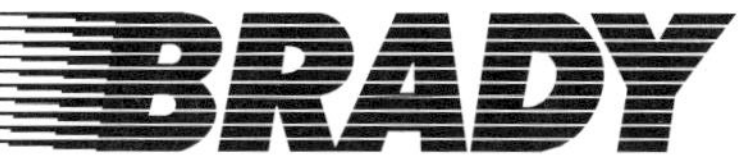

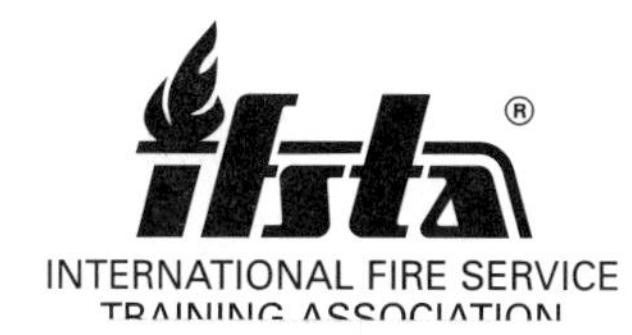

WORKBOOK

FIRE SERVICE FIRST RESPONDER

Daniel Limmer

Michael Grill

Validated by: The International Fire Service Training Association

IFSTA Senior Editor: Michael A. Wieder

Medical Editor
Edward T. Dickinson, MD, NREMT-P, FACEP

Brady/Prentice Hall Health
Upper Saddle River, NJ 07458

Reviewer:

Our thanks to Jo Anne Schultz for her review of material and for the valuable suggestions offered.

Jo Anne Schultz, B.A., NREMT-P

Paramedic, Lifestar Ambulance, Inc., Salisbury, MD;

Level II Emergency Medical Services Instructor, Maryland Fire and Rescue Institute, University of Maryland;

Paramedic Instructor, Maryland Institute of Emergency Medical Services Systems, University of Maryland;

ACLS, BTLS, and PALS Instructor

Publisher: *Julie Alexander*

Acquisitions Editor: *Laura Edwards*

Managing Development Editor: *Lois Berlowitz*

Director of Manufacturing and Production:
Bruce Johnson

Managing Production Editor: *Patrick Walsh*

Senior Production Manager: *Ilene Sanford*

Production Liaison: *Julie Boddorf*

Project Editor: *Josephine Cepeda*

Marketing Manager: *Tiffany Price*

Editorial Assistant: *Jeanne Molenaar*

Production and Composition: *Navta Associates*

Printer/Binder: *The Banta Company*

Notice on Care Procedures

It is the intent of the authors and publisher that this workbook be used as part of a formal First Responder education program taught by qualified instructors and supervised by a licensed physician. The procedures described in this workbook are based upon consultation with First Responder and medical authorities. The authors and publisher have taken care to make certain that these procedures reflect currently accepted clinical practice; however, they cannot be considered absolute recommendations.

The material in this workbook contains the most current information available at the time of publication. However, federal, state, and local guidelines concerning clinical practices, including, without limitation, those governing infection control and universal precautions, change rapidly. The reader should note, therefore, that new regulations may require changes in some procedures.

It is the responsibility of the reader to familiarize himself or herself with the policies and procedures set by federal, state, and local agencies as well as the institution or agency where the reader is employed. The authors and the publisher of this workbook disclaim any liability, loss, or risk resulting directly or indirectly from the suggested procedures and theory, from any undetected errors, or from the reader's misunderstanding of the text. It is the reader's responsibility to stay informed of any new changes or recommendations made by any federal, state, and local agency as well as by his or her employing institution or agency.

Prentice-Hall International (UK) Limited, *London*
Prentice-Hall of Australia Pty. Limited, *Sydney*
Prentice-Hall Canada, Inc., *Toronto*
Prentice-Hall Hispanoamericana, S.A., *Mexico*
Prentice-Hall of India Private Limited, *New Delhi*
Prentice-Hall of Japan, Inc., *Tokyo*
Prentice-Hall Singapore Pte. Ltd.
Editora Prentice-Hall do Brasil, Ltda., *Rio de Janeiro*

Contents

Chapter	1	Introduction to the EMS System	1
Chapter	2	Scene Safety and the Well-Being of the First Responder	5
Chapter	3	Legal and Ethical Issues	10
Chapter	4	The Human Body	15
Chapter	5	Airway	22
Chapter	6	Circulation	34
Chapter	7	Automated External Defibrillation	41
Chapter	8	Scene Size-Up	45
Chapter	9	Patient Assessment	52
Chapter	10	Cardiac and Respiratory Emergencies	65
Chapter	11	Other Common Medical Complaints	70
Chapter	12	Environmental Emergencies	78
Chapter	13	Psychological Emergencies and Crisis Intervention	83
Chapter	14	Bleeding and Shock	87
Chapter	15	Traumatic Injuries	93
Chapter	16	Burn Emergencies	101
Chapter	17	Musculoskeletal Emergencies	106
Chapter	18	Injuries to the Head, Neck, and Spine	112
Chapter	19	Childbirth	120
Chapter	20	Infants and Children	127
Chapter	21	Lifting and Moving Patients	134
Chapter	22	Multiple-Casualty Incidents and Incident Management	138
Chapter	23	EMS Operations	143
Chapter	24	Hazardous Materials	147
Chapter	25	Fireground Rehabilitation	151
Chapter	26	EMS Rescue Operations	154
		Appendix	159
		Answer Key	171

Introduction to the EMS System

KEY IDEAS

This chapter provides an overview of the EMS system and the roles and responsibilities of the Fire Service First Responder in the EMS system. Key ideas include the following:

◆ The EMS system is a network of resources linked together for the purpose of providing emergency care and transport to victims of sudden illness and injury.

◆ The public has access to the EMS system through 9-1-1 and non-9-1-1 phone numbers.

◆ There are four levels of EMS training: First Responder, EMT-Basic, EMT-Intermediate, and EMT-Paramedic.

◆ The First Responder is the first person with emergency medical training on the scene of a sudden injury or illness.

◆ First Responders are the designated agents of the medical director, who is the physician responsible for out-of-hospital emergency medical care.

1. The emergency medical services (EMS) system is organized to:
   a. provide care to victims of sudden illness or injury.
   b. deny non-emergency personnel access to the scene.
   c. coordinate extrication and rescue operations.
   d. upgrade 9-1-1 phone systems all over the United States.

2. The National Highway Traffic Safety Administration recommends that every EMS system include 10 basic components. Write a brief description of each component:

   a. Regulation and policy:

   b. Resources management:

   c. Human resources and training:

   d. Transportation:

   e. Facilities:

   f. Communications:

   g. Public information and education:

   h. Medical oversight:

   i. Trauma systems:

   j. Evaluation:

3. There are two general systems by which the public can access EMS. They are 9-1-1 and non-9-1-1 systems.

_______ True

_______ False

4. List the four levels of out-of-hospital care providers.

a.

b.

c.

d.

5. What is your role as a First Responder? List eight tasks you should be able to perform.

a.

b.

c.

d.

e.

f.

g.

h.

6. The EMS medical director is responsible for providing guidance to all emergency care and rescue personnel.

_______ True

_______ False

7. Write an example for each type of medical control listed below.

a. Direct medical control:

b. Indirect medical control:

8. Maintaining a clean, professional appearance is nice but not a realistic goal for a fire service First Responder.

_______ True

_______ False

9. It is the fire service First Responder's responsibility to meet the standard of care with all patients, no matter their gender, age, culture, or socioeconomic background.

_______ True

_______ False

ON SCENE: First On Scene

Read this scenario and answer the questions that follow. Focus on your role/responsibilities as a First Responder.

After your engine crew responded to a fire alarm at the mall, it was determined that a group of kids pulled the alarm and ran out of the mall. As you and your crew prepare to leave, several people run out of a restaurant in the mall and yell for help. They tell you that the patient, Mr. Gianelli, must be having a heart attack. They say he cannot breathe well and is clutching his chest and neck. When you determine that it is safe to do so, you leave your vehicle, enter the restaurant, and approach Mr. Gianelli.

10. Should you act on the bystander information that Mr. Gianelli is having a heart attack? Explain your answer.

At Mr. Gianelli's side, you assess that he is awake, that he cannot speak or breathe, and that this happened while eating steak and laughing. Your partner performs a Heimlich maneuver on Mr. Gianelli, immediately expelling the bit of food that was blocking his airway. Mr. Gianelli can now breathe. His voice is very hoarse.

11. What are your roles/responsibilities now? Name at least three.

12. The EMTs arrive to continue patient care and transport. What are your roles/responsibilities now? Name at least three.

Scene Safety and the Well-Being of the First Responder

KEY IDEAS

This chapter outlines the basic steps you should take to maintain your well-being. It discusses how to anticipate and handle the emotional aspects of emergencies. It also introduces you to scene safety, including how to protect yourself against infection. Key ideas are as follows:

◆ Stress related to EMS work can have a negative affect on First Responders. Be aware of the warning signs. Lifestyle changes—including keeping physically fit and maintaining a balance between work and family—can help you deal with stress effectively.

◆ Critical incident stress requires aggressive and immediate management. One way to meet that need is through a critical incident stress debriefing, a process by which a team of peer counselors and mental health professionals help rescuers deal with their feelings.

◆ Death and dying are inherent parts of emergency medical care. When your patient is dying, you must care for his or her emotional needs as well as the injury or illness. If the patient dies suddenly, help the family or bystanders deal with their grief.

◆ The five stages of the grieving process are denial, anger, bargaining, depression, and acceptance.

◆ Another way First Responders protect themselves in the field is by preventing infection by disease. In order to do that successfully, you must practice a strict form of infection control—body substance isolation (BSI)—with all patients. You also must clean, disinfect, or sterilize your equipment properly. Also follow your physician's orders in regard to immunizations.

◆ It is imperative that you do not fall victim to the same problems that affect your patients. Therefore, do not enter the scene of an emergency until you have determined it is safe to do so. If the scene is unsafe, make it safe before you enter.

1. Identify the items below that describe high-stress situations.
   a. A patient in your care stops breathing.
   b. A hit-and-run involves an eight-year-old boy.
   c. You hear that a coworker has died on the job.
   d. You suspect physical abuse of a patient in your care.
   e. A two-car collision results in injury to four adults.
   f. A factory worker just had part of his hand amputated.
   g. You hear loud, angry voices in the apartment to which you were called.

2. Dying patients—and those close to them—experience what is called the "grieving process." This process includes five stages, which are:
   a. anger, acceptance, sorrow, shock, despair.
   b. shock, silence, acceptance, anger, mourning.
   c. denial, rage, blame, forgiveness, acceptance.
   d. denial, anger, bargaining, depression, acceptance.

3. Dealing with chronic stress may require a First Responder to make some lifestyle changes. List four examples.

   a.

   b.

   c.

   d.

4. Any event that causes unusually strong emotions, which interfere with your ability to function either during an emergency or later, is called a:
   a. burnout.
   b. mental breakdown.
   c. critical incident.
   d. crisis of conscience.

5. One CISM technique is called "defusing." It is _______ than a debriefing.
   a. shorter and less formal
   b. longer and more formal
   c. shorter and more formal
   d. longer and less formal

6. A critical incident stress debriefing is usually held _______ the incident.
   a. 30 to 45 minutes after
   b. 30 to 45 minutes before
   c. 24 to 72 hours before
   d. 24 to 72 hours after

7. List six circumstances for which a First Responder would access CISM.

   a.

   b.

   c.

   d.

   e.

   f.

8. Which one of the following is NOT true of hepatitis B?
   a. It directly affects the liver.
   b. It can last for months, and it can be fatal.
   c. It is contracted through intimate contact only.
   d. An infected person may not know he or she has it.

9. When you are caring for a patient who might have tuberculosis, protect yourself against infection by:
   a. wearing an OSHA-approved respirator.
   b. avoiding any kind of artificial ventilation.
   c. turning your face away when the patient coughs.
   d. having contact only with the patient's clothing.

10. Transmission of HIV, the AIDS virus, requires intimate contact with the body fluids of an infected person. That means infection may occur in all of the following circumstances EXCEPT which one?
   a. changing an infected baby's diaper
   b. using infected blood in a transfusion
   c. injecting an infected needle into your skin
   d. sharing a warm drink with an infected person
   e. sexual contact involving the exchange of semen

11. The single most important thing you can do to prevent the spread of infection is to:
   a. get vaccinations and booster shots.
   b. wash your hands after caring for a patient.
   c. wear gloves with all patients no matter what.
   d. clean, disinfect, or sterilize your equipment.

12. The term "body substance isolation" refers to a strict form of infection control in which you assume that:
   a. where there's smoke there's fire.
   b. only blood can transmit fatal diseases.
   c. all patients who seem to be ill are ill.
   d. all blood and body fluids are infectious.

13. *ON SCENE* ◆ Describe the personal protective equipment appropriate for each of the following emergencies.

a. An unresponsive elderly man who is lying on a bed wet with urine.

b. A 16-year-old girl has been stabbed in her thigh. The blood is spurting out with force.

c. A 24-year-old male who is complaining of a painful, swollen ankle after tripping over a curb. No blood or other body fluids are present.

d. A 72-year-old woman on her living room floor who is not breathing and has no pulse.

e. A six-year-old with a shallow two-inch cut in his lower leg. A moderate amount of bleeding is present. The blood is oozing, rather than spurting.

14. *ON SCENE* ◆ Listed below are descriptions of three emergency scenes. Decide whether or not you would enter each one. Write "yes" or "no" in the space provided.

_______ **a.** You happen across an auto wreck and find two moderately injured patients trapped in a sedan. Beside the car is a downed power line.

_______ **b.** You are out one Saturday night catching a show at a nightclub when a fight breaks out just outside the front entrance. A woman screams that somebody has been stabbed. You step outside to find a large group of people gathered a short distance away. There is much screaming and shouting. The patient appears to be at the center of this group.

_______ **c.** The assailant has reportedly fled, and law enforcement officers state that they have secured the scene. They want you to look at the assault victim.

◆ ON SCENE: The AIDS Patient

Read this scenario and answer the questions that follow. Focus on strategies you can use to protect yourself and your coworkers from infectious exposure.

It's late on a Tuesday night, when you receive a call for a "man down" at a residence. Since you know that a paramedic ambulance has to come from a neighboring company, you decide to respond to the call in your private vehicle. You arrive at the scene and note that two other responders' units are parked on the street. You enter the home and find them assessing the patient in a back bedroom. The patient is 42 years old. He states that he was diagnosed with AIDS 15 months ago and was recently prescribed some medication that has been making him nauseous. This evening he threw up four times, and then may have passed out. He states that his vomit looked "a little bloody." He is pale and sweaty. Small amounts of vomit cling to his bathrobe. He also states that he is moderately short of breath, a problem associated with a recent "flu."

15. What specific sources of infectious exposure are you concerned about with this patient?

16. What personal protective gear will you wear when managing this patient?

As you begin to assist the other First Responders, you notice that one of them is not wearing protective gear. You have the opportunity to question her about this a short while later, and she states, "Look, I know that this guy has AIDS, but it's not like there's blood everywhere. I'm watching where I put my hands, so relax."

17. Critique her argument. Do you agree with her rationale? Disagree? Explain your answer.

18. You assist paramedics in transporting this patient to the hospital. En route, he vomits twice more, and you see it contains a small amount of blood. After turning the patient over to the emergency department team, what steps would you then take to eliminate possible contamination?

Legal and Ethical Issues

KEY IDEAS

This chapter describes your scope of practice and what it means to have a duty to act. It defines patient consent and explains advance directives. It also gives you an overview of various other legal issues that will affect you in the field. Key ideas include the following:

◆ First Responders must keep their practice within the scope of care as defined by the state.

◆ Among a First Responder's ethical responsibilities is to serve the physical and emotional needs of the patient with respect for human dignity and with no regard to nationality, race, sex, creed, or status.

◆ Before providing emergency care to any patient, you must determine the patient's competence and get either expressed or implied consent.

◆ A competent adult has the right to refuse treatment or to withdraw from treatment for him- or herself or for his or her child. Follow state law and local protocols in regard to advance directives.

◆ As a First Responder, you have a duty to act, or a legal obligation to provide care to a patient who needs it and consents to it. If there is a breach of duty, you could be charged with abandonment or negligence.

◆ A patient's history, condition, and emergency care are confidential. You must have a written form signed by the patient or legal guardian before you can release this information, unless you are required by law to share it.

◆ When you are called to a potential crime scene, the police must be notified. Do not enter a crime scene until it has been secured by the police and they tell you it is safe to do so. Once on scene, your priority is patient care. However, take all necessary precautions to preserve any potential evidence.

◆ Special reporting situations in your state may include reporting child, elderly, or spouse abuse; injury that is the result of a crime including sexual assault; and infectious disease exposure.

CONTENT REVIEW

1. As a First Responder, you are allowed to perform only certain defined skills. These skills are called your:
   a. duty to act.
   b. scope of care.
   c. standard of care.
   d. ethical responsibilities.

2. A competent adult is one who is:
   a. any person over the age of 18 or 21.
   b. lucid and able to make an informed decision.
   c. married, a parent, or a member of the armed forces.
   d. seriously ill or injured, which could affect judgment.

3. In order for consent to be valid, the patient must be _____ and the consent must be _____ .
   a. alert, understood
   b. informed, written
   c. competent, informed
   d. persuaded, expressed

4. Whose responsibility is it to make sure the patient understands the First Responder's plan for emergency care, including the risks?
   a. First Responder
   b. patient's lawyer
   c. patient's physician
   d. EMS medical director

5. As a First Responder, how might you go about getting a responsive, competent adult's expressed consent?

6. ***ON SCENE*** ◆ You arrive at a scene where you find a 22-year-old woman who has apparently overdosed on heroin. She is unresponsive. You begin to initiate treatment based on the idea of _______ consent.

   a. actual
   b. substituted
   c. implied
   d. mandatory

7. ***ON SCENE*** ◆ You are at the scene of a terminally ill patient who has gone into respiratory arrest in your presence. The patient's daughter arrives and insists that you withhold treatment. How should you proceed? Explain your answer.

8. If a First Responder forces emergency medical care on a patient who refuses it, the First Responder may be charged with:

   a. assault and battery.
   b. abandonment and assault.
   c. battery and attempted rape.
   d. negligence and breach of duty.

9. List six actions you should take before leaving the scene of a moderately injured adult patient who has refused your treatment.

   a.

   b.

   c.

   d.

   e.

   f.

10. The term _______ is defined as terminating care of a patient without making sure that care will continue at the same level or higher.

    a. negligence
    b. abandonment
    c. assault
    d. battery

11. If a First Responder's care deviates from the accepted standard of care and results in further injury to the patient, the First Responder may be guilty of:
    a. negligence.
    b. abandonment.
    c. assault.
    d. battery.

12. A medical identification tag is meant to inform health care workers of:
    a. the preference for private over public hospitals.
    b. physical characteristics such as a limp or stutter.
    c. a medical condition such as an allergy or diabetes.
    d. the patient's medical insurance company ID number.

13. *ON SCENE* ◆ A fire service First Responder assists other firefighters in carrying a woman away from a fire to safety. The woman's clothes are still smoldering. Very quickly, the First Responder realizes this patient needs more help than he can provide and tells the officer in charge to call for the paramedics. Does the First Responder have a duty to act while he waits for the paramedics to arrive? Explain your answer.

14. *ON SCENE* ◆ Jake works in a small chemical plant. He is also one of three employees who were trained as on-site First Responders. One day on the way to work, Jake spots a car crash along the highway. Does he have a duty to act? Explain your answer.

15. In general, ______ includes the patient's history, condition, and emergency care.
    a. assault and battery
    b. preservation of evidence
    c. confidential information
    d. the public's right to know

Read this scenario and answer the questions that follow. Focus on the rights that adult patients have regarding consent to medical care, as well as the obligation of First Responders to encourage patients to go to the hospital should they appear to need medical care.

It is two o'clock in the morning. You are working on the engine at your volunteer fire department when you are paged out to respond to a possible heart attack. You arrive to find an elderly patient, Mr. Boyd, sitting on the edge of his bed. During your initial assessment, you notice that he appears to be slightly sweaty and pale. He tells you that he had a bout of chest pain that felt the same as the heart attack he had one year ago. He took three of his nitroglycerin pills, which relieved the pain. He says he is feeling much better and does not wish to go to the emergency room. The paramedic ambulance, which is coming from the next town, has yet to arrive. His wife says he really needs to be taken to the emergency room and that his last heart attack "almost killed him."

16. Does this patient need to go to the hospital? Explain your answer.

17. Describe two strategies you might use to convince the patient that he should go with the paramedics to the hospital.

    a.

    b.

Mr. Boyd is still refusing treatment and transport even after the paramedics arrive and complete their assessment. By now his skin has dried and he appears less pale. He states that he is pain-free, has no other symptoms, and that he will follow up with his doctor in the morning. His vital signs appear stable, and he is fully alert. The paramedics have by now become frustrated with Mr. Boyd's reluctance to go to the hospital with them. In exasperation, they tell him that if he will not go voluntarily, they will force him to go against his will. A wrestling match ensues, with Mr. Boyd finally restrained on a wheeled stretcher.

18. Do you agree with the paramedics' strategy? What rights does an alert adult patient have to refuse treatment and transport?

The Human Body

KEY IDEAS

This chapter introduces you to basic anatomy and physiology. Key ideas include the following:

◆ An understanding of key anatomical and topographic terms is important for describing a patient's position, as well as the location of injuries and other physical findings.

◆ The three main body cavities are the thoracic, abdominal, and pelvic.

◆ Major body systems are the skeletal, muscular, circulatory, respiratory, digestive, urinary, endocrine, reproductive, nervous, and integument (skin) systems.

◆ Understanding the anatomy and physiology of these systems is critical if you are to understand your patients' injuries and illnesses.

CONTENT REVIEW

1. Match the following terms of position to their correct descriptions.

anatomical •	• face up, lying on the back
lateral recumbent •	• face down, lying on the stomach
prone •	• standing, arms down, palms out
supine •	• lying on the side

2. The injury to the patient's abdomen was _______ to the bottom of the sternum.
   a. inferior
   b. superior
   c. anterior
   d. posterior

3. The _______ thorax includes the chest and abdomen.
   a. inferior
   b. superior
   c. anterior
   d. posterior

4. The patient suffered a _______ injury, which was less than an eighth of an inch deep (4 mm).
   a. deep
   b. medial
   c. lateral
   d. superficial

5. The entrance wound from the bullet was _______ to the left nipple. It almost looked as though it had entered through the patient's left side.
   a. deep
   b. medial
   c. lateral
   d. superficial

6. The bruise to the patient's chest was _______ to the right nipple, along the right border of the sternum.
   a. deep
   b. medial
   c. lateral
   d. superficial

7. The patient was experiencing _______ neck pain where the back of her neck impacted the headrest during a collision.
   a. posterior
   b. anterior
   c. proximal
   d. distal

8. The fracture to the patient's leg appeared to be to the lower thigh, just _______ to the knee.
   a. posterior
   b. anterior
   c. proximal
   d. distal

9. The patient had a forearm fracture. She was able to feel a strong pulse _______ to the injury, at the patient's wrist.
   a. posterior
   b. anterior
   c. proximal
   d. distal

10. The swelling to the patient's face was isolated to the cheek, just _______ to the left eye.
   a. inferior
   b. superior
   c. anterior
   d. posterior

11. Complete the puzzle.

ACROSS

  3. A bone of the forearm
  4. Shoulder blade
  5. A bone of the upper leg
  6. Eye socket
  8. _______ spine, or neck
 10. Part of the spine formed by five fused vertebrae
 11. A bone of the forearm
 12. A bone of the lower leg
 13. A bone of the upper arm

DOWN

  1. Kneecap
  2. The lower back
  7. A bone of the lower leg
  8. Bones that form top, back, and sides of skull
  9. Hipbone

12. The abdominal cavity is separated from the thoracic cavity by the:
  a. ribs.
  b. lungs.
  c. stomach.
  d. diaphragm.

13. The lungs and heart are found in the _______ cavity.
  a. pelvic
  b. cranial
  c. thoracic
  d. abdominal

14. The intestines are found in the _______ cavity.
  a. pelvic
  b. cranial
  c. thoracic
  d. abdominal

15. The _______ cavity is bounded by the lower part of the spine, hip bones, and pubis.
  a. pelvic
  b. cranial
  c. thoracic
  d. abdominal

16. The largest part of the liver is located in the _______ quadrant of the abdomen.
  a. left upper
  b. left lower
  c. right upper
  d. right lower

17. The left kidney is located in the ______ quadrant of the abdomen.
   a. left upper
   b. left lower
   c. right upper
   d. right lower

18. The spleen is located in the ______ quadrant of the abdomen.
   a. left upper
   b. left lower
   c. right upper
   d. right lower

19. Ligaments connect:
   a. bone to bone.
   b. muscle to bone.
   c. different layers of muscle.
   d. internal organs to bone and muscle.

20. The side impact from the car crash broke the patient's upper arm, or:
   a. ulna.
   b. radius.
   c. humerus.
   d. patella.

21. The ______ is made up of the top, back, and sides of the skull.
   a. femur
   b. cranium
   c. mandible
   d. iliac crest

22. The ______ is made up of 33 bones called vertebrae.
   a. coccyx
   b. lumbar spine
   c. spinal column
   d. xiphoid process

23. The bones that make up the shoulder girdle are the:
   a. clavicle and scapula.
   b. humerus and radius.
   c. ileum and ischium.
   d. tibia and fibula.

24. Explain the difference between smooth and skeletal muscles.

25. The passage of air into and out of the lungs is called:
   a. exhalation.
   b. expiration.
   c. respiration.
   d. inspiration.

26. All of the following are related to breathing and the respiratory system EXCEPT:
   a. alveoli.
   b. bronchi.
   c. larynx.
   d. pharynx.
   e. trachea.
   f. ventricle.
   g. epiglottis.
   h. oropharynx.
   i. bronchiole.
   j. nasopharynx.

27. The area posterior to the mouth and nose is called the:
   a. pharynx.
   b. diaphragm.
   c. costal cartilage.
   d. left main bronchus.

28. After air enters the mouth and nose, it passes through the _______ , down through the _______ , and into the _______ .
   a. pharynx, larynx, trachea.
   b. trachea, larynx, pharynx.
   c. pharynx, nasopharynx, oropharynx.
   d. oropharynx, nasopharynx, pharynx.

29. Use words from the list below to complete the sentences. Note that not all the words in the list are used and some may be used more than once.

smaller	harder	more
larger	softer	less

   a. Every part of an infant or a child's airway is _______________ than an adult's.

   b. In children, the tongue takes up _______________ space than an adult's.

   c. In infants, the tongue is _______________ likely to cause a blocked airway.

   d. The trachea of an infant or a child is _______________ flexible, narrower, and _______________ than the trachea of an adult.

30. The smallest vessels through which the exchange of fluid, oxygen, and carbon dioxide takes place are called:
   a. alveoli.
   b. venules.
   c. arterioles.
   d. capillaries.

31. Draw a line to connect each arterial pulse point to its correct location.

   carotid •   • upper arm

   femoral •   • wrist

   brachial •   • thigh

   radial •   • neck

32. The organs of the digestive system include all of the following EXCEPT:
   a. pancreas.
   b. epidermis.
   c. esophagus.
   d. alimentary tract.

33. Which system consists of two kidneys, two ureters, one urinary bladder, and one urethra?
   a. urinary
   b. endocrine
   c. digestive
   d. reproductive

34. Which of the following is NOT true of the endocrine system?
   a. It influences behavior.
   b. It stimulates breathing.
   c. It influences reproduction.
   d. It affects physical strength.

35. Which system includes ovaries and fallopian tubes?
   a. urinary
   b. endocrine
   c. digestive
   d. reproductive

Read the scenario below and answer the questions that follow. Focus on how knowledge of anatomy and physiology can help you to manage patients in the field.

You and your engine crew have just responded to an unhelmeted bicyclist who was hit by a car and thrown onto the pavement. She is complaining of pain to the upper right quadrant of her abdomen and to her right chest. She has suffered huge scrapes to her side and abdomen. She has a large bruise on her forehead. In addition, she does not remember the collision and continues to repeat the same confused questions over and over. Her breathing appears rapid and labored.

36. Which abdominal organs may be injured?

37. An injury to which system is probably causing this patient to be confused?

38. Her rapid breathing is quite noticeable. It is obvious to you that this patient has a problem with her respiratory system. Would you treat this problem before or after treating her abdominal pain and scrapes to her skin? Explain your answer.

39. You examine the patient further and find that she has a leg injury. It appears that the large bone of her lower leg is fractured just below the knee. The fracture has caused the lower leg to be turned away from the midline of her body. Using the terms described on pages 52-53 of your text, describe the position of the leg and its injuries.

CHAPTER 5

Airway

Airway and breathing management are the most important tasks performed by First Responders. Key ideas include the following:

◆ The first priority in any emergency is to establish and maintain a patient's airway. Without an open airway or adequate respirations, a patient will die within minutes.

◆ Accurate and efficient patient assessment will provide you with the information you need to determine whether or not your patient requires airway or breathing assistance.

◆ A patient's airway may need to be opened using either the head-tilt/chin-lift or the jaw-thrust maneuver.

◆ Breathing is assessed using the look, listen, and feel method.

◆ Artificial ventilation, or rescue breathing, is the procedure used to ventilate patients who are not breathing or who are breathing inadequately.

◆ First Responders must learn to assess and treat patients with partial and complete airway obstructions. Different methods are used for treating infant, child, and adult patients.

◆ Aids to resuscitation also can be used to help patients with airway or breathing problems. They include airway adjuncts such as oropharyngeal and nasopharyngeal airways, suction units, oxygen-administration equipment, and bag-valve-mask devices.

1. Trace the flow of air through the respiratory tract during inhalation. Number the following items 1–6 in the correct sequence.

   _______ alveoli

   _______ pharynx

   _______ mouth and nose

   _______ trachea and larnyx

   _______ bronchi and lungs

   _______ epiglottis

2. Circle the letter next to the item(s) that describe what happens during inhalation.
   a. The muscles between the ribs contract.
   b. Air pressure inside the chest decreases.
   c. The patient's diaphragm falls and flattens.
   d. The size of the thoracic cavity decreases.

3. Circle the letter next to the item(s) that describe what happens during exhalation.
   a. The patient's diaphragm rises.
   b. The patient's chest muscles relax.
   c. The size of the thoracic cavity increases.
   d. Air pressure inside the lungs increases.

4. Fill in the missing information from the table below.

Normal Breathing Rates	
Adult	_______ to _______ breaths per minute
Child	_______ to _______ breaths per minute
Infant	_______ to _______ breaths per minute

5. The chest wall is softer in infants than in adults. So, _______ can alert you to respiratory distress in an infant.
   a. the epiglottis
   b. excessive movement
   c. wheezing and stridor
   d. air pressure inside the chest

6. Why can tipping an infant's head back or allowing the head to fall forward be a problem?
   a. It will make breathing effortless.
   b. The positions can close the trachea.
   c. The diaphragm will fall and flatten.
   d. Because the chest wall is softer in infants.

7. The tongue of an infant or a child takes up more space than in an adult. It therefore can:
   a. use a back blow immediately.
   b. block the airway more easily.
   c. keep the trachea open more often.
   d. loosen the cricoid cartilage quickly.

8. When you perform a head-tilt/chin-lift on an infant or a child, you should:
   a. hyperextend only the head.
   b. hyperextend the head and neck.
   c. tilt the head back only slightly.
   d. tilt the head back as far as possible.

9. Describe how to perform a head-tilt/chin-lift maneuver on an adult patient.

10. The head-tilt/chin-lift and jaw-thrust maneuvers:
    a. align the nasal passages with the throat.
    b. align the pharynx with the epiglottis.
    c. lift the tongue away from the throat.
    d. flex the windpipe at a 90° angle.

11. *ON SCENE* ◆ Your patient fell six feet (2 m) onto concrete from a ladder. Which of the
    following methods would you use to open her airway?
    a. recovery position
    b. jaw-thrust maneuver
    c. head-neck/in-line move
    d. head-tilt/chin-lift maneuver

12. *ON SCENE* ◆ You are at the scene of a patient who was found unresponsive in his bed.
    His wife insists that there has been no fall or other blow that may have caused a recent
    injury. To open the patient's airway, use a:
    a. recovery position.
    b. jaw-thrust maneuver.
    c. head-neck/in-line move.
    d. head-tilt/chin-lift maneuver.

13. The oropharyngeal airway is used to maintain the airway of an unresponsive patient who
has a gag reflex.

_______ True

_______ False

14. To determine the proper size oropharyngeal airway for your patient, measure it from the:
    a. lips to the base of the tongue.
    b. corner of the nose to the top of the ear.
    c. tip of the nose to the tip of the earlobe.
    d. corner of the lip to the angle of the jaw.

15. Briefly describe how to insert an oropharyngeal airway in an adult patient.

16. To use an oropharyngeal airway in an infant or a child, insert it:
    a. tip side up.
    b. flange side first.
    c. in its upright position.
    d. in an upside-down position.

17. The nasopharyngeal airway is used to maintain the airway of a patient who has a
gag reflex.

_______ True

_______ False

18. To determine the proper size nasopharyngeal airway for your patient, measure it from the:
    a. lips to the base of the tongue.
    b. corner of the nose to the top of the ear.
    c. tip of the nose to the tip of the earlobe.
    d. corner of the lip to the angle of the jaw.

19. Briefly describe how to insert a nasopharyngeal airway in an adult patient.

20. If during insertion of a nasopharyngeal airway you meet resistance, you should try:
    a. finger sweeps and suctioning.
    b. an oropharyngeal airway instead.
    c. inserting it from the other end.
    d. inserting it into the other nostril.

21. ***ON SCENE*** ◆ You have just inserted a nasopharyngeal airway into your patient's nostril. As you reassess the patient's condition, you find that he is breathing spontaneously but you can detect no air movement through the tube. What should you do?
    a. Remove the adjunct airway immediately.
    b. Insert an oropharyngeal airway immediately.
    c. Place the patient in the recovery position.
    d. Rotate the adjunct airway from side to side.

22. To help maintain an open airway in an unresponsive patient who has not been injured, is breathing adequately, and has a pulse:
    a. insert an airway adjunct.
    b. suspect gastric distention.
    c. place him or her in a recovery position.
    d. perform a finger sweep and suction.

23. Describe the procedure for using a suctioning device. Number the following items 1–5 in the correct sequence.

    _______ Take BSI precautions.

    _______ Turn on the suction unit.

    _______ Apply the suction catheter from side to side.

    _______ Insert the catheter to the base of the tongue.

    _______ Select the correct type catheter for your patient.

24. Use suctioning for up to _______ seconds in an infant, _______ seconds for a child, and _______ seconds for an adult.
    a. 2, 2, 2
    b. 3, 6, 9
    c. 5, 10, 15
    d. 7, 13, 21

25. Briefly describe in three steps how you can determine the presence of breathing in an unresponsive patient.

    a.

    b.

    c.

26. An ominous sign of inadequate breathing is a slower than normal breathing rate. Fill in the table below.

	Inadequate Breathing
Adult	Less than _______ respirations per minute
Child	Less than _______ respirations per minute
Infant	Less than _______ respirations per minute

27. Circle the letters next to the signs and symptoms of inadequate breathing.
   a. Drowsiness, confusion
   b. Flaring of the nostrils
   c. Increased effort to breathe
   d. Inadequate chest wall motion
   e. Seesaw motion of abdomen and chest
   f. 18 breaths per minute in an infant
   g. 15 breaths per minute in a child
   h. 12 breaths per minute in an adult
   i. Gasping and grunting sounds with breathing
   j. Unequal rise and fall of the sides of the chest
   k. Slow heart rate accompanied by slow breathing rate
   l. Retractions between the ribs or above the collarbone
   m. Bluish discoloration of the skin or mucous membranes

28. Briefly describe four indications of adequate artificial ventilations.

   a.

   b.

   c.

   d.

29. Briefly describe three indications of inadequate artificial ventilations.

   a.

   b.

   c.

30. Mouth-to-mask ventilation is preferred over the mouth-to-mouth and mouth-to-barrier device techniques. Circle the letters beside the reasons why.
   a. It frees your hands for other emergency care needs.
   b. It eliminates exposure to the patient's exhaled air.
   c. It allows you to deliver ventilations of adequate force.
   d. It prevents direct contact with a patient's body fluids.

31. You must maintain a jaw-thrust maneuver during artificial ventilation of a patient with suspected spinal injury.

_______ True

_______ False

32. List the basic steps of mouth-to-mask ventilation.

33. Fill in the missing information from the table below.

	Artificial Ventilation Rates		
Adult	——— breaths per minute at	——— to	——— seconds each.
Child	——— breaths per minute at	——— to	——— seconds each.
Infant	——— breaths per minute at	——— to	——— seconds each.
Newborn	——— breaths per minute at	——— to	——— seconds each.

34. *ON SCENE* ◆ You attempt to ventilate an unresponsive patient for the first time and find that you are unable to force air into the lungs. Your next step should be to:
  a. check for a foreign body airway obstruction.
  b. reposition the patient's head and try again.
  c. suction the patient's airway for 15 seconds.
  d. insert a nasopharyngeal airway and try again.

35. A patient who has had all or part of the _______ surgically removed has had a laryngectomy.
  a. thorax
  b. epiglottis
  c. lungs
  d. larnyx

36. A ——— is a permanent opening that connects the trachea directly to the front of the neck in a laryngectomy patient.

   a. stoma
   b. larynx
   c. stamen
   d. stollen

37. ***ON SCENE*** ◆ You are at the scene of a near-drowning of a ten-month-old baby. The patient has a pulse but is not breathing. Your crew members are inexperienced at managing such a young patient, and they need your help. Respond to the following concerns.

   a. "How should we open the airway? Same way as an adult's?"

   b. "I'm having a really hard time fitting my mouth around the baby's mouth. It's so small. What should I do?"

   c. "How often should I breathe for this patient?"

38. Which of the following is NOT a recommended method for reducing gastric distention in an infant or a child?

   a. Gently press down on the patient's abdomen.
   b. Breathe slowly when ventilating the patient.
   c. Avoid ventilating the patient too forcefully.
   d. Allow the patient to fully exhale between ventilations.

39. The following list includes safety precautions you should take when you handle oxygen cylinders. Circle the letters next to the statements that are true.

   a. Never store cylinders below 125°F (57.7°C).
   b. Never "crack" a tank with a wrench.
   c. Never allow smoking near an oxygen cylinder.
   d. Never place your body over the cylinder valve.
   e. Always stand a cylinder upright near a patient.
   f. Always keep cylinder valves closed when not in use.
   g. Keep cylinders secured, especially during transport.
   h. All cylinders must have the correct regulator valves.
   i. Never allow combustible materials to touch the cylinder.

40. The most common cause of an airway obstruction in an unresponsive patient is:
   a. food.
   b. dentures.
   c. the tongue.
   d. aspirated vomit.

41. The treatment for a partial airway obstruction in an adult with good air exchange includes:
   a. encouraging the patient to cough up the foreign body.
   b. delivering five back blows for each abdominal thrust.
   c. having the patient get into a supine position.
   d. dislodging the object with finger sweeps.

42. When relieving a complete airway obstruction in a responsive adult patient, you should alternate back blows with abdominal thrusts.

   ______ True

   ______ False

43. Describe the four basic steps for clearing a foreign body airway obstruction in a responsive adult.

   a.

   b.

   c.

   d.

44. *ON SCENE* ◆ You are managing a 17-year-old patient with an airway obstruction. After you apply several abdominal thrusts, the patient falls unconscious to the ground. What should you do next?
   a. Perform five more abdominal thrusts.
   b. Attempt chest thrusts as you would for CPR.
   c. Place the patient in the recovery position.
   d. Perform a tongue-jaw lift and a finger sweep.

45. All of the following patients have a foreign body airway obstruction. Which one(s) should receive the recommended treatment for an adult?
    a. one-year-old
    b. three-year-old
    c. five-year-old
    d. seven-year-old
    e. nine-year-old
    f. eleven-year-old
    g. thirteen-year-old

46. Suspect an infection in an infant who has sudden onset of respiratory distress with coughing, gagging, stridor, or wheezing, especially when food or small items are found near the patient.

    _______ True

    _______ False

47. *ON SCENE* ◆ Your eight-month-old patient has a partial foreign body airway obstruction with poor air exchange. You may attempt to relieve the obstruction with back blows and chest thrusts.

    _______ True

    _______ False

48. After you determine that you must relieve a foreign body airway obstruction in an infant, you should proceed as follows. (Write the numerals 1–5 to show the correct sequence of steps.)

    _______ Deliver up to five back blows.

    _______ Deliver up to five chest thrusts.

    _______ Position your hand on the infant's sternum.

    _______ Turn the infant face up, with head lower than body.

    _______ Straddle the infant face down over one of your arms.

49. If you are alone, and you are unable to open the airway of an infant who is found unresponsive, you must activate the EMS system within:
    a. 15 seconds.
    b. 30 seconds.
    c. 1 minute.
    d. 3 minutes.

50. *ON SCENE* ◆ Your patient is an unresponsive infant with a foreign body airway obstruction. Write the numerals 1–5 to describe the correct sequence of steps you should take.

_______ Deliver five back blows.

_______ Deliver five chest thrusts.

_______ Perform a tongue-jaw lift.

_______ Open the airway, and deliver breaths.

_______ If you see the object, perform a finger sweep.

ON SCENE: A Drowning Victim

Read this scenario and answer the questions that follow. Focus on correctly assessing the patient's airway and breathing status and providing the appropriate airway and ventilation interventions. Watch the patient for status changes.

You are working day shift when your engine crew is dispatched to assist paramedics on the call that you have always dreaded: a pediatric drowning. You arrive on scene—a suburban residence—well before the ambulance, gather your equipment, and run around to the backyard pool. There you are greeted by three adults. They are crowded around the limp body of a two-year-old, who is lying by the side of the pool. They are screaming, crying, and frantically yelling at you to hurry. As you approach the child, Gracie, you learn that she fell into the pool without striking her head, neck, or back. She was submerged for one or two minutes before being pulled out of the water by her mother.

You move to Gracie's side and note that she is unresponsive and blue. Gracie's mother is nearly sitting on top of you as she screams and cries. Your partner, John, shouts something to you as he approaches, but you are unable to hear him over the din.

51. What should be your first action in this situation?

52. One of the adults yells at you, "Do something! You need to breathe for her! She's not breathing!" Do you agree that this should be your first step? Explain your answer.

53. You determine that you need to breathe for Gracie. Number the following actions 1–3 to place the steps in the correct order.

______ Ventilate at a rate of 20 breaths per minute.

______ Deliver two slow breaths.

______ Determine if ventilations are adequate.

54. Gracie's stomach appears to have gotten slightly distended. What steps can you take to stop this problem from continuing?

55. Gracie suddenly vomits. What should you do?

56. After ventilating Gracie for two to three minutes, you notice that her color is improving dramatically. She begins moving her limbs, and her eyelids begin to flutter and twitch. Your next step should be to:

CHAPTER 6

Circulation

Heart disease kills many people each year. Patients who are in cardiac arrest require immediate CPR and early advanced care if they are to have any chance of surviving. This chapter focuses on recognizing patients in cardiac arrest and correctly applying CPR. Key ideas include the following:

◆ Patients in cardiac arrest need immediate CPR followed by advanced medical care, including defibrillation (shocking the heart) within eight to ten minutes.

◆ CPR helps to oxygenate and circulate the blood until advanced care can be given. Any delay in performing CPR reduces the chance that the patient will survive.

◆ Before providing CPR to your patient, you must first establish unresponsiveness, breathlessness, and pulselessness.

◆ You may stop CPR only if you are exhausted and unable to continue, if you have turned your patient over to another trained rescuer or the hospital staff, if the patient is resuscitated, or if the patient has been declared dead by a proper authority.

1. Check your understanding of the heart by reading the clues and unscrambling the words.

   a. The heart lies in the chest between the ______.   GULNS

   b. It is protected in front by the ribs and ______.   MUNRETS

   c. It is like a ______-______ pump.   DISWETOD

   d. The ______ side receives oxygenated blood.   FELT

   e. The ______ side receives blood from the body.   THIRG

   f. Blood is kept under ______ by its pumping action.   SERRUPES

   g. The ______ is a sign of the pressure exerted with each contraction.   SPLEU

2. Read the clues and unscramble the words that relate to the pulse.

   a. The pulse is felt where a large ______ lies over a bone close to the skin.   ERRATY

   b. It is felt most easily at the ______ artery.   DOARICT

   c. The ______ pulse can be felt in the underside of the upper arm.   AAIRCLBH

   d. Palpate the ______ pulse first when the patient is unresponsive.   AAILRD

3. The "chain of survival" includes four links. List them.

   a.

   b.

   c.

   d.

4. List the four conditions under which CPR may be discontinued.

   a.

   b.

   c.

   d.

5. To determine pulselessness in an adult patient, assess the _______ pulse point.
   a. pedis
   b. radial
   c. brachial
   d. carotid

6. To be able to position your hands properly for CPR, you should know the related anatomy. Label the illustration below. Write on the lines provided.

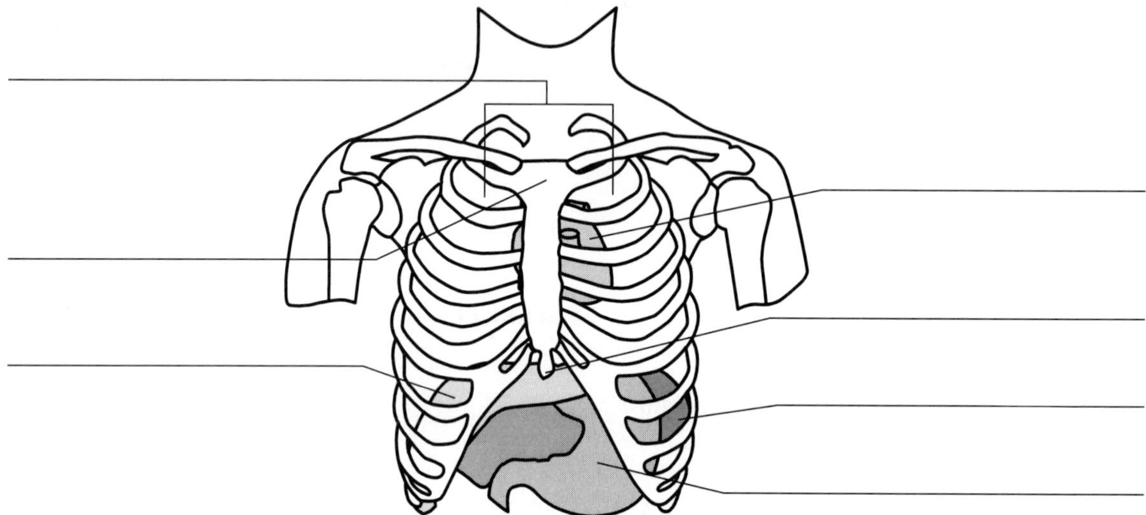

7. For you to properly perform CPR, the patient must be in a _______ position.
   a. prone
   b. supine
   c. recovery
   d. semi-sitting

8. To properly perform CPR, the patient must be on a _______ surface.
   a. hard, flat
   b. soft, flat
   c. soft, tilted
   d. hard, tilted

9. Before you may begin chest compressions, you always must determine that your patient is:

   a.

   b.

   c.

10. You will perform one-rescuer CPR on the following patients. Fill in the compression-to-breath ratio for each one.
   a. 10-year-old:
   b. 18-year-old:
   c. 3-month-old:
   d. 4-year-old:

11. You will perform one-rescuer CPR on the following patients. For each one, write in the correct hand description and position from the list.

heel of one hand   on lower half of sternum
two hands   on top third of sternum
two or three fingers   on top half of sternum

a. 5-month-old:

b. 7-year-old:

c. 71-year-old:

d. 36-year-old:

12. Fill in the chart below with the correct compression rate and depth (in inches or millimeters) for each patient.

	Infant	Child	Adult
Rate	—— per minute	—— per minute	—— per minute
Depth	—— to ——	—— to ——	—— to ——

13. Number the following actions 1–7 to correctly order the sequence of steps for adult CPR.

_______ Uncover your patient's chest.

_______ Get in position beside the patient.

_______ Thrust down and depress the sternum.

_______ Position your hands and your shoulders.

_______ Position the patient on a firm, flat surface.

_______ Locate the xiphoid process and the compression site.

_______ Completely release pressure to allow blood to flow back into the heart.

14. *ON SCENE* ◆ You are observing another First Responder perform adult CPR. You notice that he is determining his hand position by placing the heel of one hand directly over the xiphoid process. He then places his other hand on top of the first and begins compressions. Do you agree with this hand placement? Disagree? Explain your answer.

15. *ON SCENE* ◆ You observe another First Responder using jerky, jabbing movements while performing chest compressions. You believe that she needs to perform compressions more smoothly. Why? Explain your answer.

16. Describe the differences between one- and two-person CPR by filling in the chart below.

	One-Rescuer CPR	Two-Rescuer CPR
Ratio of compressions to ventilations	——— : ———	——— : ———
Check pulse after:	——— minute(s)	——— minute(s)

17. Your class is reviewing the time rule for interrupting CPR. One of the students states, "CPR should only be stopped for five seconds." Is this always possible? Give your student an example of a time he or she may need to stop CPR for more than five seconds.

18. List three injuries that can occur when CPR is performed.

a.

b.

c.

19. To determine pulselessness in an infant, assess the _______ pulse point.
a. pedis
b. radial
c. brachial
d. carotid

20. To determine pulselessness in a child, assess the _______ pulse point.
a. pedis
b. radial
c. brachial
d. carotid

21. According to AHA guidelines, if you are alone, you must attempt to resuscitate an infant or a child for three minutes before activating the EMS system.

_______ True

_______ False

22. The correct compression site for an infant is _______ an imaginary line between the nipples.
a. one finger-width above
b. one finger-width below
c. two finger-widths above
d. two finger-widths below

23. *ON SCENE* ◆ You have found Mr. Smith, a 65-year-old man, to be pulseless and breathless. When you begin compressions, you hear and feel a crunch. What should you do next? Why?

Read this scenario and answer the questions that follow. Focus on the steps necessary to assess a patient and to provide CPR.

Your engine crew is in a local grocery store doing a preplan when you hear crashing noises and screams for help. Running towards the commotion, you find a 70-year-old male patient who has collapsed from an apparent heart attack. You find the bystander administering CPR amidst a pile of overturned canned goods, the patient's up-ended cart, and a pressing mass of onlookers.

24. What should your first action be?

25. If the person providing CPR needs to be relieved, what must you do?

26. But this person does not want to be relieved right away. So you observe. He is compressing the patient's chest with his hands placed on the patient's sternum in line with the patient's nipples. He is depressing the patient's chest about one inch (25 mm) at a rate of 60 compressions per minute. Critique his CPR method and offer suggestions if necessary.

Automated External Defibrillation

Early defibrillation is necessary to the cardiac-arrest patient's survival. In order to get it to the patient early enough, as many people as possible must be able to perform this life-saving skill. This chapter provides an overview. Key ideas include the following:

◆ Defibrillation by First Responders is indicated for an adult who is unresponsive, breathless, and pulseless.

◆ Defibrillation is the definitive treatment for certain heart rhythms. CPR maintains a patient until the defibrillator can be applied.

◆ The operator of an automated or semi-automated defibrillator must follow safety guidelines.

◆ Always treat the patient, not the machine. This means assessing the patient and also reassessing after each intervention, such as a shock or movement.

◆ Post-resuscitation care is needed to monitor return of pulses, make sure the patient is breathing, and note any changes in the patient's condition.

1. What is defibrillation?

2. The letters "AED" stand for ______ defibrillation.
   a. automated external
   b. anatomical external
   c. automated electrical
   d. automatic electronic

3. *ON SCENE* ◆ A seven-year-old complained of her chest hurting, and then she collapsed. You have determined that she is unresponsive, breathless, and pulseless. Her airway is open. The paramedics will arrive in approximately two minutes. Should you start CPR or apply the AED? Why?

4. *ON SCENE* ◆ As your partner applies AED pads to the chest of an elderly woman, she tells him she is very afraid of the machine. He reassures her and tells her that her pulse is very slow and the AED will help her. He prevents everyone from touching the patient and presses the AED's "analyze" button. The machine advises a shock. Should this patient be shocked? Explain.

5. Could you use an AED on the following patients? Write "yes" or "no" beside each one.

   ______ **a.** A 12-year-old girl who weighs 85 pounds.

   ______ **b.** A 10-year-old boy who weighs 105 pounds.

   ______ **c.** A 32-year-old man who weighs 265 pounds.

   ______ **d.** A 14-year-old girl who weighs 112 pounds.

6. Explain why defibrillation should be attempted before CPR if the device is immediately available and responders trained in both AED use and CPR are present.

7. **ON SCENE** ◆ You are called to a cardiac-arrest patient with CPR in progress. When you arrive on scene with your AED ready to go, you find the patient is still unresponsive, breathless, and pulseless. Your next task is to:
   a. turn on the AED power.
   b. deliver a shock from the AED.
   c. apply the AED's adhesive pads to the patient.
   d. stop CPR and instruct everyone to clear the patient.

8. What should you do when the AED advises a shock? Number the following steps 1–7 to correctly order the steps.

   _______ Deliver the first shock.

   _______ Check the patient's pulse.

   _______ If you are advised, deliver a third shock.

   _______ If you are advised, deliver a second shock.

   _______ Wait until the AED reanalyzes the heart rhythm.

   _______ Wait until the AED reanalyzes the heart rhythm.

   _______ If there is no pulse, perform CPR for one minute.

9. Which of the following statements is correct?
   a. A non-working AED could be cause for legal action against your agency.
   b. AEDs need to be checked once a year according to the manufacturer's instructions.
   c. AEDs are simple devices and require no special care.
   d. AEDs only work after special drugs are given.

Read this scenario and answer the questions that follow. Focus on how to use an AED properly.

Your engine crew is en route to the station after fighting a long, hot house fire. You see a crowd gathered at a corner and, as you get closer, you see someone lying on the sidewalk. The driver stops the engine, and once you determine that it is safe to approach, you find two bystanders performing good CPR. Your partner assesses the patient while you set up the AED. The patient continues to be unresponsive, breathless, and pulseless.

10. When you open the patient's shirt, you find a nitroglycerin patch on the right upper chest wall. What should you do next?

11. You have attached the AED's adhesive pads to the patient's chest. The AED indicates that the patient should be shocked. What safety precaution should you take before pressing the "shock" button?

12. After the second shock is administered to your patient, the AED advises you to check the patient's pulse. You detect one. However, the patient is still breathless. What should you do now?

13. After three minutes of rescue breathing, your patient is breathing on his own at a rate of 20 times per minute. He has adequate chest rise, but he remains unresponsive without a gag reflex. At this point, what three things should you do?

    a.

    b.

    c.

Scene Size-Up

KEY IDEAS

This chapter focuses on the safety of people on scene, identifying the mechanism of injury or nature of illness, and determining the necessary additional resources. Key ideas include the following:

◆ First Responders must ensure their own safety first. This involves planning, continued observation, and appropriate reaction to danger.

◆ Before entering the scene of an emergency, the First Responder must size it up for hazards and clues to the sequence of events.

◆ First Responders must use personal protective equipment appropriate to each call.

◆ Emergency medical care of a trauma patient depends on the pattern and extent of injury. The mechanism of injury can suggest what types of injuries occurred to the patient.

◆ It is part of scene size-up to determine and call for the appropriate resources needed on scene. Do this before you begin patient care.

1. Give two examples of how you can plan ahead to stay safe at an emergency scene.

   a.

   b.

2. Decide whether or not each of the following is a sign of danger at an emergency scene. If it is, give a reason why.

   a. You witness two people arguing.

   b. There is evidence of alcohol use.

   c. There is absolute silence.

3. When you find danger at an emergency scene, there are three actions you should take. They are:

   a.

   b.

   c.

4. A "medical patient" is a patient who is _______________________________________.

5. A "trauma patient" is a patient who is _______________________________________.

6. The "mechanism of injury" refers to the:
   a. patient's chief complaint.
   b. forces that caused an injury.
   c. mechanical advantage of the body.
   d. chronic condition the patient may have.

7. The "mechanism of injury" can NOT tell you:
   a. what injuries the patient may have.
   b. if the patient was ill before injury.
   c. how serious the patient's injuries may be.
   d. what patterns of injury you should suspect.

8. Compare the patterns of injuries associated with the pathways of motion listed below.

   Up-and-over:

   Down-and-under:

9. *ON SCENE* ◆ Two cars involved in a head-on collision were traveling about 40 mph (64 km/h). The driver of a late-model sedan was wearing a lap and shoulder belt, and the car's air bag deployed on impact. His headrest was up. The driver of an old pickup truck was wearing only a lap belt. The seats of the truck have no headrests. As you approach the vehicles, you note major front-end damage to both. List the injuries you suspect each driver may suffer.

   Driver of the sedan:

   Driver of the pickup:

10. *ON SCENE* ◆ You arrive at the scene of a two-car collision. What injuries should you
    suspect in the driver whose car was broadsided?
    a. head and neck injuries
    b. chest injuries
    c. injury to the pelvis
    d. injury to the femur

11. *ON SCENE* ◆ A car is rear-ended by another vehicle, and the driver of the car does not
    have his headrest up. Immediately suspect injury to the:
    a. clavicles.
    b. carpals.
    c. cervical spine.
    d. tibia and fibula.

12. *ON SCENE* ◆ You find your patient unresponsive a few feet from her motorcycle. One
    side of the bike has large gashes in it, and the handlebar on that side has been snapped
    off. You find severe scrapes and cuts all along the patient's left side, and she has a swollen,
    deformed left lower leg. You suspect the mechanism of injury to be:
    a. ejection.
    b. head-on impact.
    c. angular impact.
    d. laying the bike down.

13. *ON SCENE* ◆ You respond to a six-year-old who has fallen 10 feet out of a tree. Her fall
    was broken by several branches. Which of the following would NOT help you to
    determine the severity of her injuries?
    a. distance of the fall
    b. body part that impacted first
    c. weight and height of the patient
    d. anything that interrupted the fall
    e. surface on which the patient landed

14. *ON SCENE* ◆ You are responding to the victim of a fall. You arrive on scene to learn that
    the patient fell 14 feet onto hard-packed dirt, landing face-down with initial contact to his
    abdomen and chest. Would you consider this a severe mechanism of injury? Why or why
    not?

15. *ON SCENE* ◆ Your patient has been stabbed. You should suspect a low-velocity injury
    that is at a site far from impact.

    _______ True

    _______ False

16. *ON SCENE* ◆ Your patient has been shot by a bullet from a handgun. You should
    suspect a high-velocity injury that affects tissues at the impact site only.

    _______ True

    _______ False

17. During the first, or primary, phase of an explosion, _______ typically causes injury.
   a. the fall onto a hard surface
   b. penetrating projectiles
   c. the pressure wave
   d. flying debris

18. Use the following clues to fill in the blanks. Then write the circled letters on the lines provided for "Scrambled Letters." Unscramble the letters to find out what safety device is important for you and the general public.

   a. A headrest will prevent the head from whipping backward after this type of impact.

   _____ _____ _____ _____

   b. An impact to the top of the head can cause this type of fracture to the cervical spine.

   _____ _____ _____ _____ _____ _____ _____ _____ _____ _____

   c. This minimizes injuries to a young child involved in a car crash.

   _____ _____ _____ _____ _____ _____ _____

   d. Seat belts and air bags help to protect motorists from serious injury in this type of collision.

   _____ _____ _____ _____ - _____ _____

   e. This abrupt stop to forward motion, such as occurs in a fall, can lead to serious injuries.

   _____ _____ _____ _____ _____ _____ _____ _____ _____ _____ _____ _____

   f. During a rollover, this may happen to an occupant who is not wearing a seat belt.

   _____ _____ _____ _____ _____ _____ _____ _____

   g. This is often called a "broadside," or "T-bone," collision.

   _____ _____ _____ _____ _____ _____ _____ _____ _____ _____

   h. This can be broken when the chest strikes the steering wheel.

   _____ _____ _____ _____ _____ _____ _____

   i. This event often results in three distinct phases, each with a typical pattern of injury.

   _____ _____ _____ _____ _____

Scrambled Letters: _____ _____ _____ _____   _____ _____ _____ _____ _____

Unscrambled Letters: _____ _____ _____ _____   _____ _____ _____ _____ _____

Read the following scenario and answer the questions that follow. Focus on the way in which the mechanisms of injury fit into the total picture.

You are responding to a vehicle collision in your rescue unit. When you arrive on scene, you can see that four cars are involved. As you begin to unload equipment, a police officer tells you the story:

A small pickup truck broke down in the middle of the roadway just over a rise. A station wagon coming over the rise at high speed rear-ended the truck. A pile-up ensued when a large sedan came upon the crash, locked its brakes, went into a sideways skid, and rolled three times. The sedan ended up over an embankment, the driver ejected. A fourth car, a foreign compact, managed to avoid the crash but slid sideways into a concrete barrier, striking the driver's side with no intrusion into the passenger space. Each car had one occupant. Each driver had taken safety precautions as follows:

- Pickup-truck driver wore a lap and shoulder belt, his headrest was up, and he had an air bag.
- Station-wagon driver wore a lap belt only and her headrest was up.
- Sedan driver had on no restraints of any kind and his headrest was down.
- Compact-car driver wore a lap and shoulder belt, her headrest was up, and she had an air bag.

19. You expect the driver of the station wagon to have taken either one of two pathways of motion. What are they?

20. Would the air bag have helped the driver of the compact car to avoid injury? Explain your answer.

21. Based on the mechanism of injury for each driver and the safety precautions each has taken, rank the four patients from most to least injured.

    a.

    b.

    c.

    d.

22. What injuries should you suspect in each of the drivers? Match the following injury patterns to the drivers.

    a. Suspect injuries to the left shoulder, left rib cage, and pelvis in the driver of the

    b. Suspect minor neck strain and a possible broken left clavicle in the driver of the

    c. Suspect lethal head and chest injuries in the driver of the

    d. Suspect major facial injuries, a broken sternum, and broken ribs in the driver of the

Patient Assessment

KEY IDEAS

This chapter focuses on gathering accurate information about the patient's condition in order to provide the appropriate care. Key ideas include the following:

◆ First Responders must assess a patient's condition quickly and accurately using a step-by-step plan. This patient assessment plan will help you focus on important concerns and establish patient care priorities. It also will help you maintain self-control in stressful situations.

◆ The First Responder's patient assessment plan consists of a scene size-up, initial assessment, physical exam, patient history, ongoing assessment, and patient hand-off.

◆ There may be instances when you are unable to complete every aspect of the patient assessment plan because of priorities, such as establishing an airway or ventilating the patient. There will also be instances where you will be able to combine steps (for example, noting a patient's level of responsiveness as you assess his or her pulse).

◆ Whenever possible, use mnemonics such as "AVPU" (levels of responsiveness), "DOTS" (what to look for during a physical exam), and "SAMPLE" (information in the patient history) to help you remember important assessment steps.

◆ Noting changes in key areas—such as level of responsiveness and vital signs—can provide valuable information about your patient to other responders and the emergency department staff.

◆ A proper patient assessment and history will help you to make sense of the patient's condition and provide quality patient care.

1. What are the six steps of the First Responder's patient assessment plan?

   a.

   b.

   c.

   d.

   e.

   f.

2. The initial assessment is the most important part of the patient assessment plan because it identifies:
   a. life-threatening problems.
   b. the patient's medical history.
   c. potential long-term disabilities.
   d. painful, swollen, or deformed limbs.

3. Put a check next to the items that are included in the initial assessment:

   _______ a. examining the pupils

   _______ b. measuring blood pressure

   _______ c. assessing the patient's ABCs

   _______ d. forming a general impression

   _______ e. conducting a head-to-toe exam

   _______ f. assessing level of responsiveness

   _______ g. updating incoming EMS units

   _______ h. the patient's chief complaint

   _______ i. taking spinal precautions

4. *ON SCENE* ◆ You are responding to a 10-year-old patient who was struck by a car traveling 30 mph (48 km/h). The patient was thrown 25 feet (8 m) onto the roadway. Number the following steps 1–7 to show the order in which they should be performed.

______ Open and assess the airway.

______ Check for serious external bleeding.

______ Update EMS, and ask for the ETA of incoming units.

______ Assess for approximate rate and rhythm of pulse.

______ Manually stabilize the patient's head and neck.

______ Introduce yourself and ask: "What happened? Where do you hurt?" Tell the patient you are there to help.

______ Assess for adequate rise and fall of the chest, ease of breathing, and adequate breathing rate.

5. *ON SCENE* ◆ You are managing a 62-year-old woman who collapsed at her office. Her airway is clear, and her respirations are 4–6 per minute and shallow. Her carotid pulse is slow and weak. Which of the following actions should you take?
   a. Do nothing because the patient's ABCs are fine.
   b. Reassess the patient every three to five minutes.
   c. Respirations are too slow. Begin artificial ventilation.
   d. Begin CPR in order to support this patient's breathing.

6. The patient's ______ is the response to the question, "Can you tell me why you called EMS today?"
   a. chief complaint
   b. mechanism of injury
   c. level of responsiveness
   d. airway and breathing status

7. The AVPU mnemonic is helpful in describing a patient's level of responsiveness. Write the description beside each letter.

   A:

   V:

   P:

   U:

8. *ON SCENE* ◆ You are assessing a patient's mental status. The patient answers all you questions but does not offer any elaboration of his own. He appears to be distracted and in distress. Using the AVPU scale, how would you describe his level of responsiveness?

9. **ON SCENE** ◆ Several ice-skaters collided, fell, and your patient was the guy on the bottom. He is responsive and, in fact, appears to be quite normal until you ask him, "What happened?" His response: "What do you mean?" Upon further questioning, you discover he does not recall the incident. Using the AVPU scale, what is this patient's level of responsiveness?

10. How would you assess the level of responsiveness in an adult whose mental status is normally altered?

11. How could you determine a two-year-old's level of responsiveness?

12. You are managing a critically injured patient who has copious amounts of blood and broken teeth blocking her airway. You should:
    a. assess the airway and then move on to assess circulation.
    b. continue to try to clear the airway until you succeed.
    c. use forceful ventilations to try to clear the airway.
    d. reassess the airway every five minutes.

13. List three signs of adequate breathing:
    a.

    b.

    c.

14. To determine inadequate breathing, look for all of the following EXCEPT:
    a. cyanosis.
    b. hemorrhaging.
    c. minimal chest rise.
    d. mental status changes.
    e. little or no air exhaled.
    f. extremely slow respirations.

15. If you determine that your patient's breathing is inadequate, you should:
    a. perform a head-to-toe exam.
    b. begin ventilating immediately.
    c. place him in a recovery position.
    d. ask bystanders if the patient was injured.

16. Generally, if your patient is a verbally responsive adult, use the _______ pulse to assess circulation.
   a. radial
   b. femoral
   c. carotid
   d. brachial

17. During the initial assessment of an unresponsive adult, use the _______ pulse to assess circulation.
   a. radial
   b. femoral
   c. carotid
   d. brachial

18. During the initial assessment, the pulse check for all infants is done at the _______ artery.
   a. radial
   b. femoral
   c. carotid
   d. brachial

19. If you find serious bleeding in your patient during the initial assessment, you should:
   a. phone or radio for help.
   b. control the blood flow immediately.
   c. provide CPR for one minute and then update EMS.
   d. reassess level of responsiveness and airway.

20. After the initial assessment of your patient, what information should you include in your update to EMS?

21. Write the numbers 1–6 to show the order in which you should perform a physical exam on an adult.

   _______ extremities

   _______ chest

   _______ head

   _______ pelvis

   _______ abdomen

   _______ neck

22. **ON SCENE** ◆ Read each scenario below. Then mark either "yes" or "no" to indicate whether or not you should perform a complete physical exam on the patient.

    ______ **a.** Your patient has fallen 15 feet (5 m) onto a concrete sidewalk.

    ______ **b.** A 36-year-old man has accidentally cut his lower arm with a broken piece of glass.

    ______ **c.** Your unresponsive patient has been found lying on a bench in the park.

23. There are three methods you should use to perform a physical exam. They are:

    a.

    b.

    c.

24. The DOTS mnemonic can help you remember the signs of injury you are looking for during a physical exam. Write what each letter stands for.

    D:

    O:

    T:

    S:

25. For which of the following findings should you stop a physical exam to administer immediate care?
    a. neck pain
    b. tenderness to the groin
    c. fracture to the lower arm
    d. open wound to the leg with minimal bleeding

26. If you were to find an open wound of the chest in your patient, you should ______ immediately.
    a. manually stabilize her head and neck
    b. apply an occlusive (airtight) dressing
    c. observe for deformities and tenderness
    d. palpate the area around it for swelling

27. To assess circulation in the lower extremities, you should palpate the ______ and ______ pulse points.
    a. dorsalis pedis, posterior tibial
    b. brachial, dorsalis tibial
    c. femoral, posterior pedis
    d. brachial, femoral

28. Vital signs include the patient's:

a.

b.

c.

d.

e.

29. More important than any one vital sign is change in vital signs over time.

_______ True

_______ False

30. A respiration consists of _______ inhalation(s) and _______ exhalation(s).
a. one-half, one-half
b. only an, not an
c. one, one
d. two, two

31. A normal adult respiratory rate is _______ breaths per minute.
a. 8–16
b. 12–20
c. 14–26
d. 15–30
e. 25–50

32. A normal respiratory rate for a child is _______ breaths per minute.
a. 8–16
b. 12–20
c. 14–26
d. 15–30
e. 25–50

33. A normal respiratory rate for an infant is _______ breaths per minute.
a. 8–16
b. 12–20
c. 14–26
d. 15–30
e. 25–50

34. To assess breathing properly, you should count the patient's respirations for _______ seconds and then multiply by _______ to get the respiratory rate.
a. 40, 1
b. 30, 2
c. 15, 3
d. 10, 4

35. A normal pulse rate for an adult is ______ per minute.
   a. 12-20
   b. 60-100
   c. 60-140
   d. 100-190

36. A normal pulse rate for two- to 10-year-olds is ______ per minute.
   a. 12-20
   b. 60-100
   c. 60-140
   d. 100-190

37. A normal pulse rate for a patient who is three months to two years old is ______ per minute.
   a. 12-20
   b. 60-100
   c. 60-140
   d. 100-190

38. If a patient's pulse rate is irregular or slow, count the beats for ______ seconds and then multiply by ______ to get an accurate reading.
   a. 40, 1
   b. 30, 2
   c. 15, 3
   d. 10, 4

39. Write what the following skin signs tell you about a patient's condition.

   a. Cool skin:

   b. Hot skin:

   c. Pale skin:

   d. Blueness:

   e. Black-and-blue mottling:

40. A reading of a patient's blood pressure can tell you:
   a. if pressure is being exerted by circulation.
   b. if the patient is an adult, child, or infant.
   c. how well pressure is being exerted in the body.
   d. how well the organs and tissues are being oxygenated.

41. Use the SAMPLE mnemonic to help you to remember important areas of questioning. Write what each letter stands for.

S:

A:

M:

P:

L:

E:

42. *ON SCENE* ◆ You are with an 81-year-old patient who is complaining of nausea, aching in all joints, weakness, and occasional dizziness. Are the patient's complaints signs or symptoms? Explain your answer.

43. *ON SCENE* ◆ You are with a 29-year-old medical patient who says he is "not feeling very well." Write two questions you might ask for the "S" part of a SAMPLE history.

44. *ON SCENE* ◆ You are waiting for the EMTs to arrive for an adult who is having trouble breathing. After you perform an initial assessment, the patient's problem appears to have eased considerably. You now are gathering a patient history. Write two questions you might ask for the "A" part of a SAMPLE history.

45. *ON SCENE* ◆ Your patient is elderly, confused, and frightened. A shop owner found her wandering in his store. She knows who she is and where she lives, but she cannot remember why she is in the store. After your initial assessment, you question her. What might you ask for the "M" part of a SAMPLE history?

46. *ON SCENE* ◆ You are with a 50-year-old patient who is having chest pain. What might you ask for the "P" part of a SAMPLE history?

47. Repeat the ongoing assessment every ______ minutes for an unstable patient and every ______ minutes for a stable one.
   a. 1, 10
   b. 5, 15
   c. 10, 20
   d. 15, 25

48. List the major elements of the patient hand-off report.

49. *ON SCENE* ◆ Joanne's patient hand-off report includes the following: "The patient's name is Pat O'Brien. He is 32 years old, and he has a painful and swollen right leg. Pat is alert with normal airway, breathing, and circulation. I've kept his leg manually stabilized in the position in which it was found for the last 10 minutes. Pat says his pain has been somewhat relieved." What information did Joanne omit from her report?

Read this scenario and answer the questions that follow. Focus specifically on the priorities of each of the major areas of patient assessment, from scene size-up through the patient hand-off report. Keep in mind that patient assessments answer the questions "What's going on with my patient? How can I help?" Continually ask yourself if the information you are gathering will help with the care of your patient's problem.

You are pulling a volunteer shift at the local firehouse late one night when you and one other First Responder are dispatched to a vehicle collision. You respond in the rescue truck and soon arrive at the scene of a single car rollover on a two-lane country road. There are no bystanders on scene. Your patient, a male in his forties, has been ejected from the car and lies in the roadway face up. As your partner quickly sets out flares to protect the scene, you confirm that there are no immediate scene dangers. Then you grab your jump kit and move to the patient's side. Your partner joins you and immediately stabilizes the patient's head and neck.

50. Your first task is to:
    a. assess airway, breathing, and circulation.
    b. inspect and palpate for any major injuries.
    c. determine if the patient has a chief complaint.
    d. find out from your dispatch the ETA of the ambulance.

51. As you kneel down beside the patient, you note that he has snoring respirations and his tongue seems to be blocking his airway. The correct way to open his airway is to:
    a. perform a head-tilt/chin-lift maneuver.
    b. perform a jaw-thrust maneuver.
    c. use the recovery position so blood and vomit can drain more easily.
    d. hold his head in a neutral, in-line position.

As you continue to assess the patient, you talk to him. He responds by calling out, speaking incoherently, and moaning. His breathing appears to be very labored and rapid. His pulse is thready, rapid, and very weak.

52. Based on this information, use the AVPU scale to describe the patient's level of responsiveness.

53. As you begin your physical exam, your patient, who had been moaning and shouting, now becomes very quiet. What should your first action be?

If you have time before the EMTs arrive, how will you perform a physical exam on this patient?
Beside each area of the body, write what you would do.

54. Head:

    D:

    O:

    T:

    S:

55. Neck:

    D:

    O:

    T:

    S:

56. Chest:

    D:

    O:

    T:

    S:

57. Abdomen:

    D:

    O:

    T:

    S:

58. Back (posterior):

    D:

    O:

    T:

    S:

59. Pelvis:

    D:

    O:

    T:

    S:

60. Extremities:

    D:

    O:

    T:

    S:

12. After you apply oxygen, you attempt to gather a patient history. List at least five questions to which you should get answers.

   a.

   b.

   c.

   d.

   e.

13. During the patient history, George becomes unresponsive. You have an automatic external defibrillator with you. At what point should you attempt to patch George into the machine? Explain your decision.

14. You determine that George is in cardiac arrest, and you begin CPR. You turn over CPR to a bystander and set up the AED. As directed by the AED, you deliver three shocks to George's heart. You are able to feel a carotid pulse, so you provide artificial ventilation until the paramedics arrive. After they take over, you give them a report. Write your hand-off report below, being sure to include your original assessment of George, his status change, and the care you provided.

CHAPTER 11

Other Common Medical Complaints

KEY IDEAS

This chapter focuses on common medical complaints other than cardiac and respiratory emergencies. These complaints include altered mental status, hyperglycemia and hypoglycemia, poisoning, stroke, seizures, and abdominal pain and distress. Key ideas include the following:

◆ First Responder care for altered mental status focuses on assessing and monitoring the patient's airway and breathing, and administering oxygen if you are allowed.

◆ First Responder emergency care for both hyperglycemia and hypoglycemia focuses on supporting the patient's airway and breathing and, if your EMS system allows, the administration of sugar.

◆ Your top priority in a poisoning emergency is the patient's airway. If EMS resources are delayed, call your regional poison control center or medical direction for instructions.

◆ First Responder emergency care for stroke focuses on maintaining the patient's airway and breathing.

◆ First Responder emergency care for seizures focuses on maintaining the patient's airway and breathing, and protecting the patient from injury.

◆ First Responder emergency care for abdominal pain consists of assuring the patient's airway and breathing, administering oxygen if possible, and staying alert for signs of shock.

1. When your patient's chief complaint is as general as "I feel weak," you should proceed with your patient assessment plan and emergency care the same as you would for any patient.

   _______ True

   _______ False

2. Identify from the list below all the possible causes of altered mental status.
   a. Decreased levels of oxygen in the blood
   b. Low blood sugar
   c. Stroke
   d. Seizures
   e. Fever
   f. Infection
   g. Poisoning
   h. Head injury
   i. Psychiatric conditions

3. **ON SCENE** ◆ It's about 2:00 in the afternoon. You and your partner spot two young men in their 20s standing in front of a bar. One of them waves you over. "Hey, this is my friend Matt. He isn't acting right. He looks drunk, but I've been with him all night and we only had a couple of beers." When you ask the patient what's wrong, he tells you he's feeling dizzy. You observe that his speech is slurred and he is staggering. How should you proceed?

4. Why is it especially important to get an accurate history from a patient with an altered mental status?

5. ***ON SCENE*** ◆ You and your partner are managing a patient with an altered mental status. The patient has a history of diabetes. You move to apply oxygen to the patient, and your partner says, "Don't bother. This guy is a diabetic. He needs sugar, not oxygen." Do you agree or disagree with this statement? Explain your answer.

6. When blood sugar is too low or too high, the body reacts. The most common reaction is:

7. Write nine signs and symptoms that could indicate a patient is suffering from hypoglycemia or hyperglycemia.

    a.

    b.

    c.

    d.

    e.

    f.

    g.

    h.

    i.

8. During scene size-up, what four observations might you make in the home of a patient who has diabetes?

    a.

    b.

    c.

    d.

9. ***ON SCENE*** ◆ You are assessing a 28-year-old man who is wearing a medallion around his neck, which says he has diabetes. He was found wandering aimlessly in the street. He is now awake but slightly confused and slow to answer your questions. List five questions you could ask this patient to gather information about his emergency.

    a.

    b.

    c.

    d.

    e.

10. List four major routes by which patients are poisoned, and give an example for each.

    a.

    b.

    c.

    d.

11. ***ON SCENE*** ◆ Your neighbor has just banged on your door, stating that her two-year-old ate a handful of mouse poison. You call 9-1-1 and run over to your neighbor's house to help. List four questions you would ask your neighbor in order to gather a good patient history about the event.

    a.

    b.

    c.

    d.

12. Common signs and symptoms of poisoning by absorption include all of the following EXCEPT:
    a. itching or irritation.
    b. redness, rash, or blisters.
    c. abdominal pain or discomfort.
    d. liquid or powder on the skin.

13. ***ON SCENE*** ◆ You have responded to a residence where it appears that a woman in her 40s has been exposed to carbon monoxide from a faulty kerosene heater. She is experiencing headaches, dizziness, and chest tightness. Since she has been removed from the house, she states that her symptoms are clearing up. Your partner says that he feels okay releasing her to follow up with her personal physician. Do you agree or disagree with this decision? Explain.

14. List three types of signs or symptoms a patient who has had a stroke might exhibit. Give an example of each one.

    a.

    b.

    c.

15. Evaluate the following statements regarding stroke and the treatment for stroke. Write "agree" or "disagree" beneath each one. If you disagree with the statement, explain.

    a. Provide the same emergency care you would provide to any patient with an altered mental status.

    b. You need not be especially alert to the patient's airway or breathing status because stroke usually affects only the limbs, speech, or facial muscles.

    c. Do not talk to the stroke patient during emergency care, especially if the patient cannot communicate. His or her inability to respond to you will only frighten the patient further.

16. Read the statements below. Which ones are NOT appropriate to make in front of a stroke patient?
   a. It looks like this patient had "the big one." Weird vital signs, paralysis on one side. Nope, Mr. Gonzalez does not look good.
   b. Mr. Gonzalez, I can see that you are having trouble speaking. I'll be able to provide you with better care if you try harder to speak more clearly.
   c. Mr. Gonzalez, I think you are having a stroke. It looks like it's pretty bad, so I'm going to take you to the hospital.
   d. Mr. Gonzalez, let's take a ride over to the hospital. I know that you're concerned about not being able to speak clearly, so I'm going to have a doctor check you out.

17. Of all causes of seizure, which one is the most common in infants and children?
   a. hypoglycemia
   b. stroke
   c. infection
   d. fever

18. The post-seizure phase is characterized by:
   a. unusual smell or flash of light that lasts a split second.
   b. unresponsiveness followed by extreme muscle rigidity.
   c. violent jerking of the arms and legs.
   d. deep sleep with gradual recovery.

19. *ON SCENE* ◆ You have responded to a man reportedly in seizure. You arrive at the entrance to an alleyway and notice a patient lying against a building, still in seizure. A witness tells you that the patient fell to the ground and struck his head when his seizure began. Number the following actions 1–6 to correctly order the steps for managing this patient.
   _______ a. Perform a head-to-toe physical exam to look for any trauma, incontinence, medical alert bracelets, etc.
   _______ b. Size up the scene. Check for hazards and any clues that might explain his seizures.
   _______ c. Protect the patient's head until the seizure stops.
   _______ d. When the seizure stops, provide manual stabilization of the patient's head and neck.
   _______ e. Attempt to gather medical history from the patient.
   _______ f. Perform an initial assessment and provide treatment as appropriate.

20. List six signs and symptoms of abdominal pain and distress.

    a.

    b.

    c.

    d.

    e.

    f.

21. *ON SCENE* ◆ When you palpate your patient's abdomen, he turns away from you and draws his knees toward his chest. What is this position called? What does it signify?

22. Check all the items listed below that refer to a proper assessment of a patient with abdominal distress.

    ______ **a.** Perform an initial assessment first.

    ______ **b.** Gather a good patient history.

    ______ **c.** Determine whether the patient is restless or quiet.

    ______ **d.** Find out if movement causes pain.

    ______ **e.** Check to see if the abdomen is distended.

    ______ **f.** Note if the patient can relax the abdominal wall.

    ______ **g.** Palpate the abdomen gently.

    ______ **h.** Examine the area of pain first.

    ______ **i.** Determine if the abdomen is rigid or soft.

    ______ **j.** Stay alert for signs of shock.

23. *ON SCENE* ◆ Your patient is suffering from abdominal pain and is complaining of feeling nauseated. If appropriate, you should place the patient in a ______ position.

    a. supine

    b. left lateral

    c. prone

    d. shock

Read the following case study and answer the questions that follow. Pay attention to the signs and symptoms that indicate this patient has experienced some type of significant brain problem.

It's dinnertime at the station. You and the rest of the volunteer fire squad are getting ready to sit down to finish off a kettle full of spaghetti when you are dispatched to a "male in his 60s, unknown medical problem." You arrive at a residence and are flagged down by the patient's wife. "John just collapsed in the kitchen," she states as you pull your equipment from the truck. "He's awake now, but he doesn't seem right. Nothing like this has ever happened before."

She tells you that John was washing his hands at the sink when he stumbled back against a counter and slid down to a sitting position. He "just stared off into space" for at least a minute. He then appeared to become somewhat aware of his surroundings, but was unable to speak or move his left side. You find John still sitting on the kitchen floor. He looks at you as you approach, but does not speak.

24. After taking BSI precautions, you should assess John's:
    a. pupils and blood pressure.
    b. carotid or radial pulse.
    c. level of responsiveness.
    d. airway and breathing.

25. As you complete your assessment of John, you find he is able to move all extremities and he has begun to speak clearly. "What happened, Grace?" he asks his wife. After his wife explains, you begin to gather a patient history. List five questions that you could ask him in order to better understand his collapse and current condition.

    a.

    b.

    c.

    d.

    e.

Environmental Emergencies

KEY IDEAS

This chapter focuses on recognizing the causes, signs and symptoms, and emergency care of heat and cold emergencies. Key ideas include the following:

◆ The human body is constantly trying to maintain its average core temperature of around 98.6°F (37°C).

◆ In the cold, the body holds onto its heat by constricting blood vessels near its surface. Also, hair erects, thickening the layer of warm air trapped near the skin. The body can produce more heat, if needed, by shivering and by producing certain hormones such as epinephrine.

◆ The body loses heat through convection, conduction, radiation, evaporation, and respiration.

◆ Cold-related emergencies include generalized hypothermia and local cold injuries. Treatment focuses on supporting the patient's ABCs and rewarming as appropriate.

◆ Heat-related emergencies include heat cramps, heat exhaustion, and heat stroke. Treatment for these emergencies focuses on supporting the patient's ABCs and cooling the patient as necessary.

1. Check your understanding of mechanisms of heat loss by reading the clues and unscrambling the words.

   a. This occurs when moving air passes over the body and carries heat away.

   NOITONCCEV

   b. This occurs when direct contact with an object carries heat away.

   CIUDONNOCT

   c. This involves the transfer of heat to an object without physical contact.

   DANATIRIO

   d. This occurs when sweat changes to vapor.

   PRATIAVOONE

   e. This occurs when cold air is inhaled and warmed air is exhaled.

   PRESTIORIAN

2. There are five stages of hypothermia. Each one can progress to the next, more serious stage. Number the stages 1–5 to show the order of worsening hypothermia.

   _______ **a.** apathy and decreased muscle function

   _______ **b.** decreased level of responsiveness

   _______ **c.** death

   _______ **d.** decreased vital signs

   _______ **e.** shivering

3. Infants and children are better able to maintain body temperature than adults are.

   _______ True

   _______ False

4. *ON SCENE* ◆ Your patient is a 35-year-old woman who was found stumbling along a hiker's trail. She is slightly disoriented and complaining of stiff joints and weakness. She appears to be clumsy, confused, and forgetful. Her skin is cold to the touch. Given this information, list five questions you would want to ask for a SAMPLE history.

   a.

   b.

   c.

   d.

   e.

5. Identify the three items that do NOT tell how to care for a patient with generalized hypothermia.
   a. Massage cold extremities gently.
   b. Comfort, calm, and reassure the patient.
   c. Have the patient sip a hot drink or hot soup.
   d. Remove the patient from the cold environment.
   e. Administer warm, humidified oxygen if possible.
   f. Allow the patient to walk to stimulate circulation.
   g. Remove wet clothing, and cover the patient with a blanket.

6. *ON SCENE* ◆ You are extricating a severely hypothermic patient from a mountainous region. As you are lifting the stretcher into the ambulance, one member of the rescue party accidentally slams the side of the stretcher. Your partner shouts, "Hey! Be more careful! What are you trying to do, kill the guy?" Why would your partner say this? Why is it so important to handle a severely hypothermic patient gently?

7. A sign of an early or superficial local cold injury is:
   a. swelling and blistering.
   b. mottled and cyanotic skin.
   c. the skin being firm to the touch.
   d. blanching when skin is touched lightly.

8. Care of a late or deep local cold injury includes all of the following EXCEPT:
   a. rewarm it by soaking in 108°F (42°C) water.
   b. cover it with a dry cloth or dressings.
   c. manually stabilize the injured extremity.
   d. monitor the patient for signs of hypothermia.

9. List five signs and symptoms of a heat-related emergency.

   a.

   b.

   c.

   d.

   e.

10. A patient with moist, pale, and normal-to-cool skin has the very serious and life-threatening condition known as heat stroke.

   _______ True

   _______ False

11. *ON SCENE* ◆ You are managing a 27-year-old runner who has dropped out of a mini-marathon after becoming dizzy and nauseous. She presents with pale, cool, and extremely wet skin, headache, weakness, and a rapid pulse. Describe the steps for treating this type of emergency.

ON SCENE: Hyperthermia at a Structure Fire

Read the scenario and answer the questions that follow. Bear in mind that hyperthermic emergencies can happen even to healthy, fit patients.

You and your crew have responded to the scene of a structure fire. It is a hot day, and you are battling a blaze that has fully engulfed a two-story home. The incident commander pulls you from firefighter duty and asks you to set up a rehab area. He points you to your first patient—a firefighter who is sitting on the tailboard of one of the fire engines. He has stripped off his turnout jacket and helmet and appears somewhat dazed.

"How are you doing?" you ask the firefighter.

He stares at you blankly for a moment. "Fine. I'm just fine." He appears quite hot.

"How about if I just check you out. Your captain seems to think you may have gotten too hot."

"No, I'm fine, really. I just need to sit for a minute. That's all."

12. How should you respond to the firefighter at this point? Why?

13. When you examine the firefighter, you find that he is very hot to the touch, with
respirations of 36, strong pulse of 120, and blood pressure at 92/76. As you complete your
exam, he vomits. As you continue to talk to him, he becomes more confused. What do you
suspect this patient to be suffering from?

14. Another firefighter looks at your patient and states, "Get Frank some water. He looks like
he could drink a gallon." Do you agree with this request? Disagree? Explain your answer.

15. List your treatment steps for this patient.

Psychological Emergencies and Crisis Intervention

This chapter provides an overview of emergency care for patients who are having behavioral and psychological emergencies. It includes discussion about drug and alcohol emergencies, as well as rape and sexual assault. Key ideas include the following:

KEY IDEAS

◆ A behavioral emergency is one in which a patient exhibits "abnormal" behavior, or behavior that is unacceptable or intolerable to the patient, family, or community.

◆ A behavioral emergency may be the result of a physical illness or injury.

◆ Psychological care of patients means that you are accepting and helpful, not critical or judgmental.

◆ Assessing your patient for a possible behavioral emergency should be part of every scene size-up.

◆ Because signs and symptoms vary so widely and are so similar to many medical conditions, the most reliable indications of a drug- or alcohol-related emergency are likely to come from the scene and the patient history.

◆ Rape and sexual assault involve both emotional and physical trauma, as well as significant legal issues. When you care for such a patient, remember that his or her coping system has already been stressed to the limit by the attack. Supporting the patient is of critical importance.

1. Read the following quotes. Write whether you "agree" or "disagree" with the way in which the fire service First Responder deals with a patient having a behavioral emergency. If you disagree, explain your answer.

   a. "Look, pal, I know that you're upset, but killing yourself over a bad relationship is not the answer. Buddy, there's always gonna be other opportunities out there. Keep your chin up."

   b. "Look, I realize that you don't think your neck is hurt. However, you need to let me check you out now. Your neck could be broken. Do you want to spend the rest of your life in a wheelchair? I'm here to help you. Don't you want help?"

   c. "Paul, I have to tell you that we will be taking you to the hospital for an evaluation. You tried to hurt yourself tonight and we need to make sure you stay safe. I understand that you disagree with us, but we agree with the police officers, and they've decided you need to go."

   d. "Trish, my name is Scott. I'm a volunteer with the local fire department. I'm just here to make sure you're okay. Do you want to talk about what happened? Did somebody hurt you? . . . Sure, I can understand that you don't want to talk about it, Trish. Can you tell me if you are hurt anywhere?"

   e. "Look, Pat, we all get mad at stuff that goes wrong in our lives. But I'm pretty sure most of us wouldn't consider busting our hand through a plate glass window just because our kids forgot to pick up cat food at the store. You need to sort of stand back and take a look at what you've done, I think."

2. ***ON SCENE*** ◆ You have arrived at the residence of a patient with a history of mental illness. His girlfriend meets you out front and tells you that "he's pretty worked up" and that he may have a weapon ("a knife or club or something"). Which two of the following would be correct responses?
   a. Wait outside the residence and call for law enforcement to respond.
   b. Do not allow the woman to reenter the house.
   c. Discreetly investigate to verify the status of the patient.
   d. Call out to the patient from a distance to verify his status.

3. The term "reasonable force" refers to the amount of force needed to:
   a. provide life-saving care.
   b. immobilize a threatening patient.
   c. restrain a patient with metal cuffs.
   d. keep a patient from injuring anyone.

4. One way to protect yourself against false accusations by a patient is to carefully and completely document everything that occurs during a call.

   _______ True

   _______ False

5. List four common signs and symptoms of a life-threatening drug- or alcohol-related emergency.

   a.

   b.

   c.

   d.

6. ***ON SCENE*** ◆ Your patient is unresponsive. You suspect this is a drug- or alcohol-related emergency. To confirm your suspicions, what should you do immediately after your initial assessment?

7. During a drug- or alcohol-related emergency, your immediate goals are to:

   a.

   b.

   c.

Read the scenario and answer the questions that follow. Remember that managing a patient can mean managing the patient's emotions as well as actual physical injuries.

It is nearly midnight on a Saturday night, and your crew has been dispatched to assist police officers at the scene of an assault. Dispatch informs you that the victim is a female who was stabbed and may have been raped. You arrive to find the scene chaotic with police officers everywhere.

You check in with the incident commander, and she tells you that your patient is a 27-year-old female who apparently met a drug dealer at the motel to purchase drugs. Instead, the dealer dragged her into the alley, raped her, and then stabbed her in her upper arm. Bleeding has stopped. The drug dealer was frightened off by the motel manager, who had heard the commotion in the alley and came to investigate.

You approach the patient, who sits huddled with a blanket wrapped around her shoulders. She is crying softly, and sits clutching herself.

8. As a First Responder, what would you say to this patient initially? Write out a few sentences.

9. You delegate the treatment of the patient's arm laceration to another First Responder. As he moves to touch the wound with some dressings, she pulls away sharply, clutching herself harder and shouting, "Don't get near me! Don't touch me!" The First Responder pulls away in alarm. How would you deal with her response? Describe at least two strategies for handling this situation.

10. Aside from the knife wound and a few minor bumps and bruises, the patient does not appear to have any other significant physical injuries. Blood loss from her stab wound is minor overall. The patient states that she does not have any major vaginal bleeding. What is your treatment plan for this patient at this point? Be specific.

Bleeding and Shock

KEY IDEAS

This chapter focuses on how to control both external and internal bleeding and how to recognize and manage shock. Key ideas include the following:

◆ Treating life-threatening bleeding takes priority over all other treatments except emergency care of the patient's airway and breathing.

◆ Emergency medical care of a patient who has external bleeding includes direct pressure, elevation, the use of pressure points, and splinting.

◆ Internal bleeding is managed by maintaining the patient's ABCs and treating for shock.

◆ Shock, or hypoperfusion, is a condition that results from the inadequate delivery of oxygenated blood to the body's tissues.

◆ Shock may progress in stages from compensatory shock to decompensated shock, and finally to irreversible shock, which is fatal.

◆ The key to effective prehospital care of the shock patient is early recognition, immediate treatment, and rapid transport to an emergency department.

1. When managing an agitated patient with a profusely bleeding head laceration, which of the following describes adequate BSI precautions?
   a. gloves and eye protection
   b. gloves only
   c. gloves and a gown
   d. gloves, gown, and eye protection

2. List the four basic methods of controlling external bleeding.

   a.

   b.

   c.

   d.

3. Which pressure points are most commonly used to control bleeding?
   a. brachial, femoral
   b. ulnar, carotid
   c. brachial, radial
   d. femoral, pedal

4. Which one of the following statements about tourniquets is NOT true?
   a. A tourniquet can be improvised from a scarf, towel, belt, or necktie.
   b. A tourniquet can completely shut off the blood supply to a limb, causing permanent disability or even loss of the limb.
   c. A tourniquet can be released once bleeding has been controlled.
   d. A tourniquet should be used only as a last resort after all other methods of bleeding control have failed.

5. The best position for a patient with a nosebleed is:
   a. lying face up with the head tilted back.
   b. sitting up with the head tilted back.
   c. lying on the right or left side.
   d. sitting up and leaning forward.

6. List five signs and symptoms of internal bleeding.

   a.

   b.

   c.

   d.

   e.

7. A fellow First Responder has approached you looking for some advice. Here is her story:

"I just helped the EMTs transport a young guy who ran his car into a telephone pole. His car was a real mess. It took us about 20 minutes to cut him out of it. He had some lacerations from all the broken glass and metal. In fact, I helped to control bleeding to his right forearm. He also said that he had neck and back pain.

Initially he looked pretty good. The weird thing was that by the time we got him extricated, he was as white as a sheet. After we immobilized him on a long backboard and loaded him in the back of the ambulance, he was breathing really fast and getting combative. The EMT was unable to get a blood pressure, and his pulse was almost too fast to count.

As we transported him with lights and siren, we applied 100% oxygen and elevated his legs. We frantically looked for any signs of trauma, but except for the lacerations and some abdominal pain, we couldn't find anything. The guy died in the ER. What do you think happened? Did we miss something?"

What happened to this patient?

8. Identify all the signs of compensatory shock listed below.
   a. mottled skin
   b. unresponsiveness
   c. normal blood pressure
   d. slightly elevated pulse rate

9. Identify all the signs of decompensated shock listed below.
   a. extreme thirst
   b. very rapid heart rate
   c. normal blood pressure
   d. major changes in mental status

10. Which two of the following statements are true about irreversible shock?
   a. It can be stopped with aggressive treatment.
   b. It leads to the destruction of major organs.
   c. It causes slightly narrowed pulse pressures.
   d. It shunts blood away from the liver and kidneys.

11. Which of the following is a late sign of shock?
   a. pale skin
   b. low blood pressure
   c. skin color changes
   d. restlessness or anxiety

12. Which of the following would be among the earliest signs and symptoms of shock?
    a. cool, moist skin
    b. low blood pressure
    c. very rapid heart rate
    d. restlessness or anxiety

13. What is First Responder emergency care of a patient who presents with signs of shock? Briefly list the steps.

◆ ON SCENE: Pedestrian–Vehicle Collision

Read this case study and answer the questions that follow. Focus on the patient's ABCs and the early recognition of shock.

A 12-year-old female named Paula rode her bike through an intersection and was struck by a car traveling 30 mph (48 km/h). She was thrown about 25 feet (7 m) onto the concrete pavement.

14. You find Paula in the middle of the intersection, surrounded by Good Samaritans. She appears to be unconscious. What will be your first action at this scene?

15. As you complete your initial assessment of Paula, you notice that she has snoring respirations at a rate of six breaths per minute. You also notice that she is bleeding profusely from a large gash just below her left groin. What will your next action be?

16. Which bleeding control measures would be most appropriate for this patient?

17. You have completed your initial assessment and have performed a quick head-to-toe exam. You found the following: Paula is responsive to pain only. She has a large bruise to her forehead, large scrapes to her left side, a laceration to her leg, and a painful, swollen, deformed right arm. Her vitals are: respirations 6, pulse 120, BP 116/72, with pale, cool, moist skin. Which two of the above findings concern you the most? Why?

18. The following is a list of tasks you complete while managing Paula. Write whether each one is a "high" or "low" priority.

__________________ **a.** Maintain Paula's airway using an appropriate airway maneuver.

__________________ **b.** Ventilate Paula with supplemental oxygen.

__________________ **c.** Try to determine Paula's previous medical history.

__________________ **d.** Cover Paula's cuts and bruises.

__________________ **e.** Determine if any on-scene bystanders witnessed the incident.

__________________ **f.** Establish that the scene is safe from hazards.

__________________ **g.** Place an ice pack on Paula's forehead bruise.

__________________ **h.** Reassess Paula's level of responsiveness every five minutes.

__________________ **i.** Inform bystanders of Paula's condition.

__________________ **j.** Determine the speed of the car that struck Paula.

Traumatic Injuries

This chapter focuses on the assessment and management of wounds. Key ideas include the following:

◆ Wounds are classified as open or closed, single or multiple. They are also classified by location.

◆ Closed wounds include contusions and clamping or crushing injuries. Open wounds include abrasions, lacerations, and penetration/puncture wounds.

◆ In general, emergency care of soft-tissue injuries includes treatment for external and internal bleeding.

◆ The basic purposes of dressings and bandages are to control bleeding, to prevent further contamination and damage to the wound, to keep the wound dry, and to immobilize the wound site.

1. Complete the crossword puzzle below.

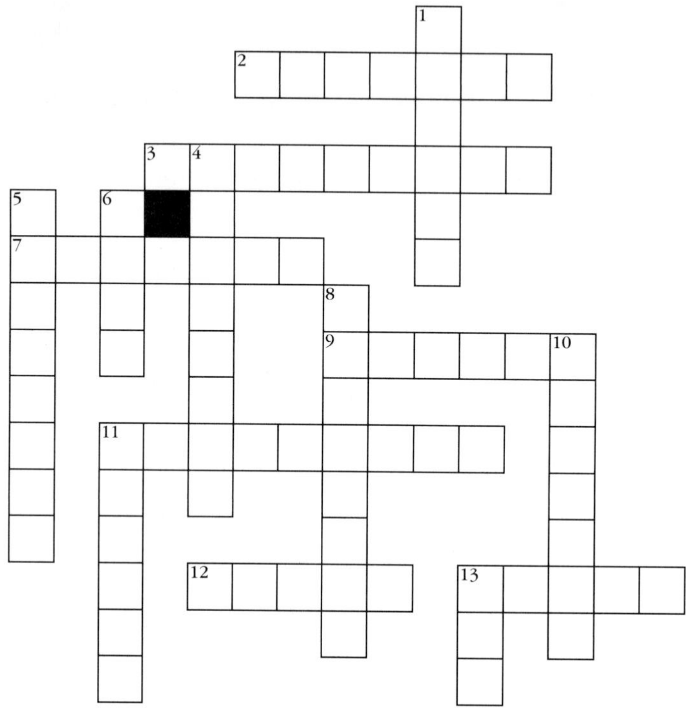

ACROSS

2. A(n) _____ object is one that is embedded in an open wound.

3. A special type of dressing used to form an airtight seal

7. Used to hold a dressing in place, create pressure, or provide support

9. A viral infection usually associated with animal bites

11. A closed soft-tissue injury characterized by swelling and pain at the injury site

12. A soft-tissue injury is also called a(n) _____ .

13. A(n) _____ dressing is a large, thick, layered pad.

DOWN

1. A hematoma is evident as a lump with _____ discoloration.

4. A(n) _____ injury is one that usually involves a finger or limb stuck in an area smaller than itself.

5. An open wound caused by scraping, rubbing, or shearing away of the epidermis

6. Use a square _____ to tie a bandage in place.

8. A sterile covering for an open wound

10. The state of being free of all microorganisms and spores

11. A triangular bandage that has been folded

13. Take _____ precautions to prevent contact with a patient's blood or body fluids.

2. ***ON SCENE*** ◆ Your patient has just been struck in the forearm by a baseball bat. Describe what the contusion might look like and how you would care for this injury.

3. Next to each mechanism of injury below, write the type of soft-tissue injury you would expect to see.

avulsion   amputation   puncture/penetration
laceration   bite   abrasion

_______________________ **a.** Patient was thrown from her bicycle and slid across the pavement.

_______________________ **b.** Patient's wound occurred when his arm slid along the jagged metal of the car frame.

_______________________ **c.** Patient suffered an injury when she stepped on a nail.

_______________________ **d.** Headliner of a car caught the patient's forehead as he was ejected.

_______________________ **e.** Toddler came screaming from the sandbox, "Fido hurt me!"

_______________________ **f.** A gang member said that he was cut with a razor blade.

_______________________ **g.** Police officers state that the assault victim was attacked with a broken whiskey bottle.

_______________________ **h.** Witnesses think the patient's finger was caught in the power planer.

_______________________ **i.** Small power sander shot a large splinter of wood at the patient's arm.

4. The steps below describe how to manage a patient with an amputation of the forearm. Write 1–10 to put the steps in the correct order.

_______ **a.** Remove clothing to expose the entire injury site.

_______ **b.** Wrap the severed part in saline-moistened, sterile gauze.

_______ **c.** Dress and bandage the stump.

_______ **d.** Administer oxygen by way of a nonrebreather mask.

_______ **e.** Assure an open airway and adequate breathing.

_______ **f.** Complete an initial assessment.

_______ **g.** Control bleeding with direct pressure and elevation.

_______ **h.** Size up the scene for hazards and the mechanism of injury.

_______ **i.** Wipe away loose particles of foreign matter from the wound.

_______ **j.** Perform an ongoing assessment until the EMTs arrive to take over care.

5. ***ON SCENE*** ◆ You are at the scene of a stabbing. A fellow First Responder turns to you and states the following: "The patient was stabbed in the back just above the scapula. It looks like there is minimal bleeding from the wound. The police found the knife, and it only has a two-inch (55 mm) blade, so this guy should be okay." Agree? Disagree? Explain.

6. ***ON SCENE*** ◆ You are caring for a patient who has a one-foot (30 cm) steel rod impaled in his abdomen. Which one of the following would NOT be an appropriate action?
   a. Manually stabilize the steel rod.
   b. Remove clothing to expose the injury site.
   c. Cut the rod to make it easier to manage.
   d. Administer oxygen by way of a nonrebreather mask.

7. Correct treatment for a patient who has a pen impaled through his cheek includes which one of the following?
   a. Stabilize the pen with bulky dressings.
   b. Cut the pen to make it a manageable size.
   c. Position the pen so it cannot occlude the airway.
   d. Remove the pen and apply bulky dressings to the wound.

8. Because significant soft-tissue injuries to the chest can allow air to flow where it should not, apply a(n) _______ dressing to all open chest wounds.
   a. occlusive
   b. pressure
   c. bulky
   d. roller

9. Open soft-tissue injuries to the neck should be sealed airtight with a(n) _______ dressing.
   a. occlusive
   b. pressure
   c. bulky
   d. roller

10. On rare occasions, you may be required to manage an evisceration. Describe how you would dress or bandage it.
   a. Replace exposed organs and cover with a thick, moist dressing.
   b. Replace exposed organs and cover with light, dry gauze.
   c. Leave exposed organs as found and cover with a thick, moist dressing.
   d. Leave exposed organs as found and cover with light, dry gauze.

11. Proper care for a patient with an avulsion to the scalp includes which one of the
following?
   a. Place the skin flap in its normal position.
   b. Fold the skin flap away from the open wound.
   c. Dress the wound exactly the way you found it.
   d. Remove the skin flap and place it on a cold pack.

12. One of the primary purposes of a dressing is to:
   a. hold a bandage in place.
   b. prevent the bandage from sticking to the wound.
   c. ensure that the wound remains sterile.
   d. prevent further contamination of the wound.

13. Which two of the following statements about bandaging are true?
   a. Make sure the bandage is sterile.
   b. Remove a patient's jewelry first.
   c. Bandages should allow air to reach the wound.
   d. Loosen bandaging if it proves to be too tight.

14. Analyze the following statements by First Responders regarding bandaging. Then write
"agree" or "disagree" beside each one. If you disagree, explain why.

   a. "My patient just told me that the bandage is too tight, but I convinced her to leave it
   the way it is so that the laceration won't start bleeding again."

   b. "The laceration is about four inches (100 mm) long on the side of the patient's foot.
   It was bleeding pretty badly when I arrived on scene, so I went ahead and covered
   up the entire foot with bandages."

   c. "I thought that the bandage on the forearm wound might be too tight, but the patient
   said it felt fine. His fingers were warm and pink, and he had a good radial pulse, so I
   left it."

   d. "My partner had covered the wound with some gauze dressings and roller bandages,
   but the edges of the wound were exposed, so I removed the bandaging and added a
   larger trauma dressing to cover the entire area."

e. "I made a pressure bandage by applying some dressings to the wound and then folding two triangular bandages into cravats and tying them tightly around the dressings."

15. *ON SCENE* ◆ The saw that Ray Gonzalez was using slipped and sliced open his thigh. He sees all the blood and is terrified. "I'm going to die!" he says in a husky whisper. You answer him:
    a. "Most people don't die from cuts like this. Just relax. It'll be okay."
    b. "You're not going to die. Now, if you had gotten cut where your femoral artery is, that would be a different story."
    c. "I'm going to help control the bleeding here. You can help me by lying back down so that I can see where to put my dressings."
    d. "It looks pretty bad, but I'll do what I can to get this bleeding under control."

16. *ON SCENE* ◆ You are still with Ray Gonzalez, the patient described above. You don gloves and then place a handful of 4×4 gauze pads on the wound. They are quickly saturated with blood. Which dressing or bandage should you apply next to this wound?
    a. more gauze pads
    b. an occlusive dressing
    c. a roller bandage
    d. a trauma dressing

17. *ON SCENE* ◆ After applying direct pressure with dressings to Mr. Gonzalez's wound for several minutes, it appears that the bleeding has slowed to a trickle. Which of the following bandaging materials would make the best pressure bandage?
    a. cravats
    b. triangular bandages
    c. roller bandages
    d. elastic bandages

Read the scenario and answer the questions that follow. Focus on the priorities for managing a soft-tissue injury. Remember your patient assessment plan.

You have just exited a transit bus on your way home from work when you hear screams. You decide which house they are coming from—the Johnsons—and trot over. Along a side walkway is an overturned bicycle and a huge splatter of blood. From the backyard you hear the strangled sobs of a child and the frantic voice of a woman, probably his mother.

You follow the trail of blood to the backyard. "Can I help?" you call out as the mother and child come into view.

"Please, please help! Danny is bleeding badly," answers the child's mother. She has taken the child to a garden hose and is dousing a large, jagged laceration with water. It is still bleeding profusely. "He cut himself on a rusty pipe at the side of the house," she explains. Her four-year-old son is frantic, sobbing, and struggling to free himself from her hold.

18. What should be your first step in getting ready to assist this child?

19. Describe your strategy for helping the child to calm down.

20. You move to turn the hose off. The mother says, "Keep the water on. He cut his leg on a rusty drain spout." What is your response?

21. You finally are able to examine the wound. It is a three-inch (75 mm) laceration, about one inch (25 mm) deep, on the front of his thigh. It stretches from midway down his thigh to his knee. Describe the location and extent of the wound. Use three of the following terms: proximal; distal; anterior; posterior; midway.

22. List the steps in controlling bleeding from this injury.

23. You have controlled the child's bleeding and have calmed both him and his mother. Paramedics have just arrived. Give them a patient hand-off report. (Information: you estimate that the child has lost perhaps 200 milliliters of blood.)

Burn Emergencies

CHAPTER 16

This chapter provides an overview of the methods of classifying burns and describes basic emergency care of burns, as well as special types of burn injuries. Key ideas include the following:

◆ Burns are complex injuries that can impair a number of the body's functions, including fluid balances, body temperature, and joint function.

◆ The severity of a burn is determined by the depth of the burn, percentage of body surface burned, location of the burn, and complicating factors.

◆ Treatment for burns focuses on stopping the source of the burning, maintaining the patient's ABCs, and covering the burned area with sterile dressings.

◆ Inhalation injuries can cause severe, life-threatening respiratory distress. In addition to respiratory burns, victims of these injuries can be poisoned by the substance that has been inhaled.

◆ Chemical burns require aggressive irrigation. All significant chemical burns should be treated as severe.

◆ The most important priority in cases of electrical burns is scene safety. Treatment focuses on maintaining the patient's ABCs and should include spinal immobilization.

1. Match the signs and symptoms to the related term.

charring •   • superficial burns

red skin and swelling •

intense pain •   • partial-thickness burns

red skin and blisters •

little or no pain •   • full-thickness burns

2. ***ON SCENE*** ◆ You are managing a patient who was burned in a grease fire. He has burns covering his entire anterior chest and abdomen, as well as his anterior left arm. Using the "rule of nines," calculate the percentage of his body that has been burned.

3. Decide if each patient has critical, moderate, or minor burns. Write your answer in the space provided.

a. A 65-year-old patient received full-thickness burns to her hands and face from hot grease.

b. A 23-year-old received superficial burns to his abdomen when he spilled a pot of boiling water.

c. A 16-year-old received partial-thickness burns to her arms and chest from hot oil after her car was hit by a truck. She also suffered a fractured arm and leg.

d. A 9-year-old was rescued from a burning residence. He has a rasping cough and soot in his nostrils.

e. A 35-year-old received partial-thickness burns to his left forearm after leaning against a hot metal surface at work.

f. A 27-year-old received a superficial burn to the back of her left hand while tending the fire in her wood stove.

4. Chemical burns should be flushed with water for a minimum of _____ minutes.
   a. 5
   b. 10
   c. 15
   d. 20

5. **ON SCENE** ◆ You have responded to a victim of a house fire who has burns and inhalation injuries. The emergency care you need to provide is described below. Number the steps 1–7 to show the correct order in which they should be performed.

   _______ **a.** Perform an initial assessment.

   _______ **b.** Determine the history of the burns.

   _______ **c.** Administer oxygen via nonrebreather mask.

   _______ **d.** Remove the patient from the source of the burn.

   _______ **e.** Stop the burning process.

   _______ **f.** Cover the burns with dry, sterile dressings.

   _______ **g.** Assess the extent and severity of the patient's burns.

6. Identify all the signs and symptoms of smoke inhalation listed below.
   a. cyanosis
   b. noisy breathing
   c. skin rash or hives
   d. shortness of breath
   e. singed nasal hairs
   f. cough or hoarseness
   g. burns to the face
   h. carbon in the sputum
   i. difficulty speaking
   j. restricted chest movement
   k. bruising of the skin
   l. puncture/penetrating wounds
   m. abrasions or lacerations

7. ***ON SCENE*** ◆ You are managing a patient who received burns to his arms and face
   following a house fire. Your partner tells you, "Remove everything on his arms and hands
   so that we can take care of his burns." He has rings on his fingers, a watch on one wrist,
   and charred clothing hanging from both arms, some of it embedded in the burns. Which
   of these items do you want to remove? Which do you want to leave alone? Why?

◆ ON SCENE: Electrocution Victim

*Read the scenario and answer the questions that follow. Remember that patients who have been
electrocuted may have extensive internal injuries and organ damage not immediately evident. Be
sure to prioritize your care to treat the patient for life-threatening injuries first.*

You arrive at a canal levy where a farmer was electrocuted by a downed power line. Bystanders
tell you that the farmer was driving his tractor near the levy when he ran into a downed power
line. He was electrocuted when he hopped off the tractor to investigate. You see that the farmer
is lying near his tractor. Members of the local fire department who arrived on scene before you
tell you that they removed the power line and it is safe to approach the patient.

8. As you cautiously move closer to the farmer, you notice that the soles of your feet begin to
   tingle. What is causing this, and what should you do?

9. The scene is now safe. You call to the farmer, but he does not respond. Based on what you
   know about electrocution injuries, what injuries are you expecting to find, and what
   equipment will you need to manage these injuries?

10. Where would you expect to find contact burns on this patient, and how will you treat them?

11. Vital signs on this patient are as follows: The farmer is unresponsive, with a pulse of 44 and respirations of 8 per minute. The farmer's blood pressure is unobtainable. You can see an ugly burn on the farmer's foot, and both of his legs appear to be fractured. Two fire department crew members are busy securing the scene from curious onlookers. Which of these findings should you manage first? Why?

Musculoskeletal Injuries

This chapter focuses on assessment and emergency care of patients with injuries to muscles, joints, and bones. Key ideas include the following:

◆ Muscle, joint, and bone injuries are some of the most common injuries First Responders will encounter. They can range from minor ankle or knee sprains to life-threatening fractures of the neck or pelvis.

◆ Accurate patient assessment and aggressive treatment of musculoskeletal injuries can prevent permanent disability and death.

◆ Since it is not possible for a First Responder to distinguish between sprains and strains or dislocations and fractures, First Responders are to treat all musculoskeletal injuries the same way.

1. An obvious injury, such as a broken leg, may actually be one of several related injuries located elsewhere in the body.

   _______ True

   _______ False

2. List five signs and symptoms of musculoskeletal injury.

   a.

   b.

   c.

   d.

   e.

3. In an emergency involving musculoskeletal injury, you should stay focused on treating the patient's life threats. Once that is done, you can turn to limb-threatening injuries.

_______ True

_______ False

4. **ON SCENE** ◆ Your patient is lying on the side of a two-lane road after falling from her bicycle. There is an open injury to her left leg half-way between the ankle and knee. What appears to be a broken bone protrudes from the wound. Number the following actions 1–8 to show the order in which they should be performed.

_______ a. Cover the open wound at the injury site.

_______ b. Assess for distal pulse, movement, and sensation.

_______ c. Complete a scene size-up.

_______ d. Splint the injured leg.

_______ e. Complete a physical examination.

_______ f. Reassess for distal pulse, movement, and sensation.

_______ g. Complete an initial assessment.

_______ h. Manually stabilize the injured leg.

5. List five reasons for splinting a musculoskeletal injury.

a.

b.

c.

d.

e.

6. **ON SCENE** ◆ The patient has an open angulated injury to the lower leg. The First Responder decides not to remove the patient's jeans before splinting in order to avoid moving the protruding bone and making the injury worse. Do you agree or disagree? If you disagree, write your reasons.

7. Complete the paragraph by filling in the missing words.

If a long bone is injured, immobilize it and the ______________ above and below it. If a

joint is injured, immobilize it and the ______________ above and below it.

8. List three problems that can be caused by improper splinting.

   a.

   b.

   c.

9. **ON SCENE** ◆ You are managing a 14-year-old patient who has a closed injury to her forearm. The bone is bent at an angle between the elbow and the wrist. You attempt to straighten it by pulling gentle traction, but she screams, "Ow! It hurts!" What should you do?

10. **ON SCENE** ◆ You and your partner are managing a patient who has fallen and presents with an elbow injury. Your partner turns to you and states, "There's no way we can leave that elbow bent like that. We need to straighten it so that extrication will be easier." What do you think? Explain your answer.

ON SCENE: Auto vs. Bridge Abutment

Read this scenario and answer the questions that follow. Focus on prioritizing the management of musculoskeletal injuries as well as on the correct technique for splinting.

You are on a Sunday drive in the country when you notice that a sedan has just crashed head-on into a concrete bridge abutment. After reporting the incident on your cellular telephone, you run over to assess the scene and the patients. The scene appears to be safe. The car has suffered severe front-end damage. The steering wheel is not bent. The windshield has been starred on the passenger side. There are three patients in the car. The status of each follows:

Patient A: 22-year-old male, driver of the car. Was restrained with a three-point seat belt. Complains of pain and swelling to his right ankle and lower left leg. Has a small bump to his forehead where he impacted the side window. Did not lose consciousness. Appears to have strong radial pulses. Skin signs appear normal. Has good distal pulses and sensation in all extremities.

Patient B: 21-year-old male, unrestrained front-seat passenger. Was hurtled against the windshield and dashboard. Presents as very combative, with a large bruise to his forehead. Has serious-looking chest injuries. Right humerus and forearm appear to be deformed. Severe pelvic pain with palpation. Has weak radial pulses. Skin is pale, cool, and moist.

Patient C: 23-year-old female, back-seat passenger. Was restrained with a three-point seat belt. Did not lose consciousness. Complains of pain and deformity to her left clavicle and wrist. Is also unable to straighten her left knee, which is swollen and painful. Has strong radial pulses. Skin is pale, warm, and dry. Has a good distal pulse and sensation in her arms. There are no pulses present at her left foot.

11. Order these patients from most (#1) to least (#3) severely injured. Explain how you arrived at your decisions.

    a. Patient A:

    b. Patient B:

    c. Patient C:

An EMT ambulance and two fire trucks arrive. A helicopter has also been dispatched. The patients are extricated and placed on long backboards. You move over to where rescuers are packaging Patient B for transport. You remember that his humerus appeared fractured during your exam, and you reach for splinting materials from an open first aid box. An EMT turns to you and says, "I appreciate your help, but that arm just gets strapped to his chest. Nothing more."

12. Why would this EMT say this? Agree? Disagree?

13. You assist with Patient C. You have already splinted her wrist and are trying to apply a sling and swathe to her injured clavicle. Every time you try to apply the sling and swathe, you move her arm slightly, causing her severe pain. "Just let me hold my left arm with my good arm," she suggests. Does this seem to be an acceptable alternative? Explain your answer.

14. Another rescuer attempts to straighten Patient C's left leg, but she screams when the responder tries to do so. Describe a splinting strategy for this injury.

15. Describe a simple technique for splinting Patient A's ankle injury.

Injuries to the Head, Neck, and Spine

This chapter focuses on spinal injuries. It covers the mechanisms of spine injuries, patient assessment, and emergency care. Key ideas include the following:

◆ Injuries to the spine can affect almost any body system. Improper handling of a spine-injured patient can kill the patient or cause permanent disability.

◆ Suspect spine injury in any patient with a head injury. If the mechanism of injury suggests a possible head injury, or if a trauma patient is unresponsive, suspect spine injury.

◆ If the mechanism of injury suggests it, assume a spine injury even if your assessment finds nothing wrong with the patient.

◆ Signs and symptoms of a spine injury can range from mild neck tenderness to paralysis and respiratory arrest.

◆ The goals of managing a spine-injured patient are to support the patient's ABCs and to stabilize his or her spine until the patient is completely immobilized.

1. **ON SCENE** ◆ You are assessing a possible head-injured patient. His level of responsiveness, as well as pulses, movement, and sensation in his extremities, appear to be normal. List six special findings that could indicate this patient has suffered a head injury.

   a.

   b.

   c.

   d.

   e.

   f.

2. **ON SCENE** ◆ You have responded to a 34-year-old male who was struck in the head with a piece of lumber at a work site. He was briefly knocked unconscious. You and your partner find the patient awake but combative and vomiting. Your partner responds, "It's probably just a concussion. How bad could it be?" Do you agree with your partner's assessment? Explain.

3. Your priorities while caring for a patient with a head injury are included in the list below. Identify all of them.
   a. controlling major bleeding
   b. protecting the patient's cervical spine
   c. maintaining an open airway and adequate breathing
   d. arranging for rapid transport to the hospital

4. List four emergencies in which your index of suspicion for spine injury should be very high.

   a.

   b.

   c.

   d.

5. If the mechanism of injury suggests it, suspect spine injury even if there are no signs or symptoms.

______ True

______ False

6. Your patient has a suspected spine injury. Immediately upon completing your ______ , stabilize her head and neck.
   a. scene size-up
   b. initial assessment
   c. physical examination
   d. ongoing assessment

7. List six signs and symptoms of a spinal injury.

   a.

   b.

   c.

   d.

   e.

   f.

8. A cervical-spine injury can result in severe breathing problems, even respiratory arrest.

______ True

______ False

9. Complete the paragraph below by filling in the missing words.

   To manually stabilize a patient's cervical spine, you must place your gloved hands

   just ___________________ the patient's ears. Then hold the patient's head

   ___________________ and ___________________ in a neutral, in-line position.

10. The word "neutral" in the term "neutral in-line position" means the head is:
    a. flexed forward and extended back.
    b. not flexed forward but extended back.
    c. flexed forward but not extended back.
    d. neither flexed forward nor extended back.

11. The word *in-line* in the term "neutral, in-line position" means the patient's:
    a. nose is in line with the chin.
    b. nose is in line with the navel.
    c. Adam's apple is in line with the navel.
    d. Adam's apple is in line with the chin.

12. If you find that the spine-injured patient's head is not in line, gently put it there, even if you feel resistance.

    _______ True

    _______ False

13. Manual stabilization must be maintained, even when the patient is immobilized on a long backboard.

    _______ True

    _______ False

14. Even the best rigid cervical immobilization devices do NOT prevent movement.

    _______ True

    _______ False

15. ***ON SCENE*** ◆ You have arrived at the scene of a side-impact motor-vehicle collision. The patient is a male in his 30s who was the driver of the car that was hit. He is complaining of neck pain. Another First Responder arrived on scene before you and applied a cervical collar to the patient's neck. You note that the patient is sitting unattended on the curb, cervical collar in place. The other First Responder is getting an incident history from bystanders. What is your opinion of the care given to this patient? Does it adequately protect his possible neck injury? Why or why not?

16. *ON SCENE* ◆ You have responded to a "man down" call. You find an intoxicated patient, James, who gives you a conflicting story. He first states that he was assaulted, struck in the head with a tire iron, and thrown to the pavement. He then states that he was really just sleeping and that his assault story actually occurred a week ago. You see what may be relatively old lacerations and bruises on his head. You find that he is unsteady on his feet (from the alcohol?) and that his grip appears quite weak. During your exam, a buddy of his, Bob, walks up and tells you that James had indeed been sleeping, and that Bob called 9-1-1 because "James was breathing kind of funny." Bob also seems fairly intoxicated. Should you take spinal precautions or not? Explain your decision.

17. *ON SCENE* ◆ You are managing a patient who has suffered a possible neck injury when diving into a pool. You arrive at her side after she has been rescued from the water. She is conscious and complains of neck pain and tingling to her arms and legs. Read the following actions. Number them 1–14 to show the order in which they should be performed.

_______ **a.** Administer high-concentration oxygen to the patient.

_______ **b.** Apply a rigid cervical immobilization device.

_______ **c.** Identify the mechanism of injury.

_______ **d.** Immobilize the patient's legs.

_______ **e.** Immobilize the patient's torso.

_______ **f.** Immobilize the patient's head.

_______ **g.** Open the airway with a jaw-thrust maneuver.

_______ **h.** Pad the spaces between the patient and the board.

_______ **i.** Perform a log roll, and place a long backboard under the patient.

_______ **j.** Perform a physical exam, including assessment of pulses, movement, and sensation in all four extremities.

_______ **k.** Reassess pulses, movement, and sensation.

_______ **l.** Reassess pulses, movement, and sensation.

_______ **m.** Stabilize the patient's head and neck.

_______ **n.** Withdraw manual stabilization.

18. Manual stabilization may be released when a patient has been properly secured to a short backboard.

_______ True

_______ False

19. The procedure called "rapid extrication" may be performed in certain emergencies. Write three examples of such emergencies.

a.

b.

c.

20. Removal of a helmet from a suspected spine-injured patient requires at least _______ rescuers.

   a. 2
   b. 3
   c. 4
   d. 5

Read the case study and answer the questions that follow. Focus on protecting the patient's spine while completing other tasks necessary to manage the patient.

You are on your three-day break from the fire department, and you are enjoying a peaceful day in the mountains when you suddenly hear screams for help coming from the direction of a nearby creek. You rush over to a small, deep pool that is popular with summer hikers and find a group of people crowded around a 16-year-old boy on a sand bar. He apparently dove into the pool and struck a small outcropping of rock with the top of his head. Fellow swimmers rescued him from the pool.

The patient, John, is lying on his back. Blood is seeping from a wound on the top of his head. One of his friends, obviously terrified, takes John by the shoulders and shakes him. "John, c'mon, get up buddy," he pleads.

"Don't touch him!" another of his friends screams. "Can't you see that he's hurt badly?"

You notice that two other ashen-faced friends are standing nearby.

21. Describe your approach to handling this situation. What might you do to get this scene under control?

22. What are your first priorities in assessing and treating John?

You find that John is awake but confused. His airway is patent. He appears to be breathing adequately, but you see that his abdomen, not his chest, moves with each breath. His pulse is 88 and strong at the wrist. His only injury appears to be the head wound. Bleeding is controlled. John is able to move his left arm slightly, which is the only extremity movement you see.

23. As you are caring for John, an onlooker says, "It looks like he can move one of his arms. That's a good sign, isn't it?" Which of the following would be the best response to this question?
    a. "He may still have a permanent spine injury. It's too early to tell."
    b. "That sure is. Keep your fingers crossed that everything's going to be okay."
    c. "Spine injuries can get worse over time. We'll have to let the doctors sort it out."
    d. "Movement is good. Since we don't know the extent of injury, we're going to hold him very still until the paramedics arrive."

By now you have completed your initial assessment and physical exam, through which John's head and neck have been manually stabilized in a neutral in-line position. Rather than speaking in confused sentences, John has become unresponsive and his eyes gaze without focusing on anything. His pulse has dropped to 44 beats per minute, and his breathing appears more labored.

24. What can you do at this point to help John?

25. "He's getting worse!" one of his friends shouts. "Let's carry him up to the road so that he'll be closer to the paramedics when they arrive." Do you agree or disagree with this plan? Explain.

26. Paramedics have arrived. Give them a brief hand-off report about John, including information about the mechanism of injury, your assessment, and your treatment.

Childbirth

| KEY IDEAS |

This chapter describes the basic anatomy of pregnancy, the stages of childbirth, and assessment and management of both the baby and mother during and after delivery. Key ideas include the following:

◆ Childbirth is a natural, normal process. However, it is physically traumatic and complications to both the baby and mother do occur, though infrequently. While emergency deliveries do occur in the field, most mothers in labor are able to deliver their babies in the hospital.

◆ Childbirth is divided into three stages of labor: dilation, expulsion, and placental.

◆ First Responders must be able to determine whether or not birth is imminent.

◆ The role of the First Responder during delivery is to help coach the mother through the delivery and then to support the mother's and baby's airway, breathing, and circulation.

◆ First Responders may at some point manage a patient experiencing pregnancy or birth complications. Most pregnancy complications can lead to shock. Pregnancy complications most commonly involve a problem with the umbilical cord or the position of the baby prior to or during delivery. Other delivery complications may involve multiple or premature births.

1. Complete the crossword puzzle.

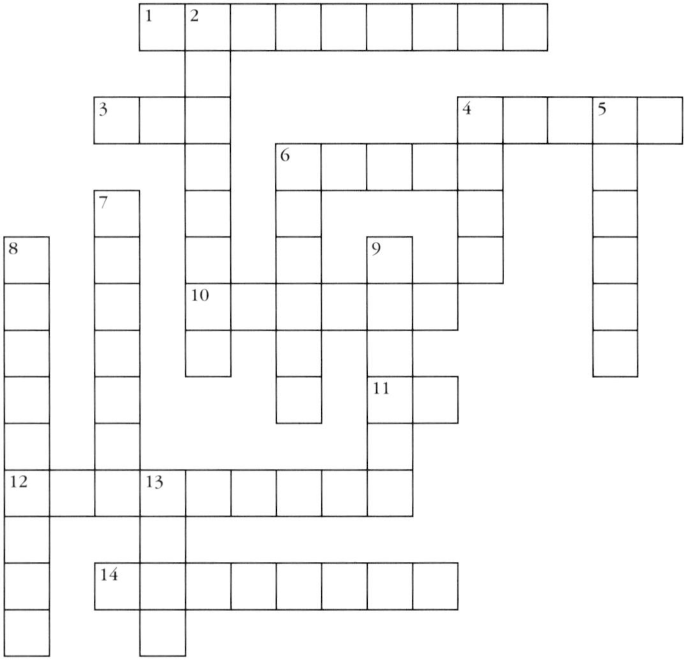

ACROSS

1. This cord may be tied or clamped after the baby is born.

3. The amniotic _______ is also called "bag of waters."

4. A premature infant may develop this condition if he or she loses any blood.

6. When the placenta is delivered, it is called the after _______ .

10. The organ that contains the developing fetus

11. A(n) _______ kit holds obstetrical equipment.

12. There may be two of these in a multiple birth.

14. When the baby's head first appears, we say the baby is _______ .

DOWN

2. You may see _______ staining of the amniotic fluid.

4. The bloody _______ may be one of the first signs of labor.

5. The neck of the uterus

6. When a baby's buttocks or feet are born first, we call it a(n) _______ birth.

7. This condition may be called "poisoning of the blood."

8. A(n) _______ cord is one that appears before the baby does.

9. Bloody show is another name for the expulsion of the _______ plug.

13. The umbilical _______ is the unborn infant's lifeline.

2. Describe the technique for measuring the length and frequency of contractions.

3. If contractions are _______ minutes apart, the mother usually has no time to be transported to a hospital.
   a. 12
   b. 7
   c. 8
   d. 2

4. List five questions you might ask an expectant mother in order to determine whether delivery is imminent.

   a.

   b.

   c.

   d.

   e.

5. List five BSI precautions you should take prior to and after delivery.

   a.

   b.

   c.

   d.

   e.

6. To prevent an explosive delivery, you should:
   a. firmly press the mother's legs together.
   b. apply firm pressure to the vaginal opening.
   c. elevate the mother's buttocks.
   d. apply very gentle pressure to the baby's head.

7. The infant emerges with the amniotic sac still intact. There is meconium staining. You break the sac and push it away from the baby's face. What should you do next?

8. Meconium staining is not a life-threatening event. Just be sure to suction out the baby's airway.

   ______ True

   ______ False

9. What should you do if after the baby's head delivers, you see that the umbilical cord is wrapped around the baby's neck?
   a. Do nothing. The baby is in no danger.
   b. Immediately cut the cord to prevent strangulation.
   c. Use two fingers to slip the cord over the baby's shoulder.
   d. Apply pressure to the baby's head to prevent it from delivering.

10. The baby has delivered, but he is not breathing. What is the first thing you should do?
   a. Suction the mouth and then the nose.
   b. Provide artificial ventilation immediately.
   c. Hold the baby by the feet and slap his buttocks.
   d. Nothing. He will breathe on his own in a few minutes.

11. The baby is still not breathing. What is the second thing you should do?
   a. Provide tactile stimulation.
   b. Provide artificial ventilation.
   c. Provide both oral and aural stimulation.
   d. Nothing. He will breathe on his own in a few minutes.

12. The baby is still not breathing. What is the third thing you should do?
   a. Suction the mouth and then the nose.
   b. Provide artificial ventilation immediately.
   c. Hold the baby by the feet and slap his buttocks.
   d. Nothing. He will breathe on his own in a few minutes.

13. Your patient has delivered both the baby and the placenta and is experiencing heavy bleeding. Management strategies for this patient include all of the following EXCEPT:
   a. Pack the inside of the vagina with gauze pads.
   b. Place sanitary napkins over the opening of the vagina.
   c. Encourage the mother to begin breastfeeding if she plans to do so.
   d. Massage the lower abdomen to help the uterus contract.

14. The primary goal(s) of managing both the mother and baby after delivery include:
   a. keeping them warm.
   b. regularly reassessing the status of their ABCs.
   c. keeping them in close contact to one another.
   d. assuring that they are both transported immediately to the hospital to be evaluated by a physician.

15. What is the proper method for maintaining perfusion in the baby when a prolapsed cord occurs?
   a. Monitor the situation carefully.
   b. Immediately clamp and cut the umbilical cord.
   c. Gently push the head off the umbilical cord.
   d. Push the umbilical cord back into the vagina.

16. *ON SCENE* ◆ You are assisting with the delivery of a baby. Your partner is ready to apply gentle pressure against the baby's head as it delivers, when he shouts, "It's a breech birth! The baby's bottom is delivering first!" The buttocks and trunk deliver quickly, but the baby's head appears to be stuck in the vaginal canal. Your next course of action should be to:
   a. rush the mother and child to the hospital.
   b. very gently pull at the baby's torso.
   c. form an airway for the baby with your fingers.
   d. slip your hand under the baby's head and pull.

Read the scenario below and answer the questions that follow. Keep in mind that labor is a natural process, not an illness or an injury.

Your crew is dispatched to assist the state police with a "delivery in progress" on a busy highway. The husband has attempted to drive his wife to the hospital—which is still about 10 minutes away—but was stopped for speeding. The woman is in labor in the backseat of the station wagon, and her frantic husband is nervously pacing by the front of the car. The state trooper is sweating bullets while trying to talk to the woman who is calling out to her husband. The trooper is very glad to see you climb off your engine.

The patient is lying sideways on the backseat with sweat pouring down her face. In between contractions, she moans softly.

17. What strategies would you use to gain control of the scene, your patient, and her husband?

18. You time the patient's contractions and find that they are 6 minutes apart, lasting about 45 seconds each. The hospital is about 10 minutes away, and traffic is relatively light. The transporting ambulance is about 3 minutes away. This is your patient's first baby. Do you want to set up to deliver the baby or arrange for the ambulance to transport her to the hospital? Explain.

19. Ten minutes have passed. The patient's "water breaks," but there is still no ambulance. Dispatch tells you that the ambulance has been caught in a heavy traffic snarl and will be delayed at least 10 more minutes. What patient exam or patient history information would help you to gauge how imminent delivery might be?

20. Your patient now tells you, "I need to push. I can't help it. I've got to push now." You check her vagina and see that the baby's head is visible. Explain what is happening.

21. The ambulance has just arrived, and so has the baby. You note that the newborn is fairly blue and limp. She is not crying. You vigorously suction, dry, and stimulate the baby, but she still remains limp and unresponsive. What is the next step in resuscitating this baby?

22. Success! The baby is now crying. She has turned from blue to pink and appears to have good muscle tone. The exuberant father wants to close the doors of the station wagon and drive his wife and child to the hospital himself. After all, he says, she is already in the car. No sense in making a mess of the ambulance, too. Do you agree or disagree with his plan? Explain your answer.

Infants and Children

KEY IDEAS

This chapter identifies emotional needs of children and parents in pediatric emergencies, describes a pediatric physical assessment, compares pediatric and adult anatomy, and identifies treatment strategies for common pediatric emergencies. Key ideas include the following:

◆ When managing an emergency involving an infant or a child, First Responders must deal compassionately with the adults who are affected by the child's illness or injury. The top priority, however, is the health and safety of the patient.

◆ Assessment of an infant or a child patient is similar to adult assessment in many ways. However, First Responders must take into account differences in anatomy and developmental characteristics when assessing an infant or a child.

◆ Pediatric patients compensate better for shock than adults do. They also tend to decompensate rapidly when their shock state becomes severe. Hypothermia will intensify the problems faced by a pediatric patient in shock.

◆ Respiratory distress is one of the most common pediatric emergencies. Treating the airway and breathing in an infant or a child is the top priority in First Responder emergency care.

◆ Most cardiac arrests in infants and children are caused by airway obstructions or respiratory arrest. Effective resuscitation depends on diligent airway and breathing management and effective CPR.

1. ***ON SCENE*** ◆ You arrive at the scene of a seizure. The patient, 18-month-old Katie, has been running a fever for the past 36 hours and reportedly had a generalized seizure lasting about 45 seconds. She is conscious and crying. Her mother is quite upset. Between sobs, the mother tells you that Katie has been undergoing some tests to determine whether she has a chronic seizure disorder.

   Your partner, impatient with the mother's tears, cuts her off and states, "Ma'am, it looks like this is a simple seizure caused by a high fever. The paramedics are here and we need to get Katie moving to the hospital." Your partner then leads the mother to the front passenger seat of the ambulance "so that the paramedics can concentrate on taking care of Katie."

   Critique his behavior. What would be an appropriate response to this parent's information and behavior?

2. The single most important care you can provide for a pediatric patient is to ensure an open airway.

   ______ True

   ______ False

3. What are five signs of early respiratory distress in infants and children?

   a.

   b.

   c.

   d.

   e.

4. If an infant's respirations are less than ______ per minute or a child's are less than ______ , assist ventilations.
   a. 20, 10
   b. 40, 20
   c. 60, 40
   d. 80, 60

5. One way to assess circulation in infants and children is by palpating a pulse. Complete the sentences below by filling in the appropriate location of those pulse points.

   a. Palpate the infant's _____________________ pulse.

   b. Palpate the unresponsive child's _____________________ or _____________________ pulse.

   c. Palpate the responsive child's _____________________ or _____________________ pulse.

6. When a pediatric patient is not breathing and has no gag reflex, a(n) _____ should be inserted to assist in maintaining an open airway.

   a. bulb syringe   **c.** nasopharyngeal airway

   b. oropharyngeal airway   **d.** tonsil-tip suction catheter

7. *ON SCENE* ◆ While caring for a five-year-old girl who has fallen feet-first about three to four feet (1 m) onto ceramic tile, a First Responder asks the parents, "How does your daughter usually respond to pain?" Explain why the First Responder asked this question.

8. Children sometimes breathe irregularly, so monitor respirations for _____ seconds to determine the rate.

   a. 15   **c.** 60

   b. 30   **d.** 75

9. For each of the following facts about pediatric anatomy, physiology, or development, list the implications for possible injuries, illness, or treatment. The first one has been completed as an example.

   a. Young children explore their world by putting objects in their mouth.
      Answer: Young children can experience foreign body airway obstruction. Always rule out foreign body aspiration with any young child complaining of difficulty breathing.

   b. Infants have proportionately larger tongues than older children and adults.

c. Children have proportionately larger heads than adults.

d. Children have much less blood volume than adults.

e. A child's skin surface is large compared to body mass.

f. Children often have extremely short necks.

10. List five signs and symptoms of shock in the pediatric patient:

a.

b.

c.

d.

e.

11. What are the most common causes of cardiac arrest in children?
    a. elevated pulse rates
    b. shock or scarlet fever
    c. noisy breathing and hypothermia
    d. airway obstruction and respiratory arrest

12. All seizures in pediatric patients should be considered potentially life-threatening.

    _______ True

    _______ False

13. **ON SCENE** ◆ You find that your patient is an infant who is breathless, pulseless, stiff, and cold in his crib. You suspect SIDS. What questions do you need to ask? List six.

    a.

    b.

    c.

    d.

    e.

    f.

14. ***ON SCENE*** ◆ The First Responder arrives on scene to find a child with injuries that raise the possibility of child abuse. The First Responder says to the parent, "You need to know that I think you have abused your child, and I'm going to report you to the hospital staff and local law enforcement." Do you think this statement was appropriate? Why or why not?

◆ ON SCENE: Shortness of Breath in a Kindergarten Class

Read the scenario and answer the questions that follow. Remember that infants and children require different levels of explanation about what is happening to their bodies and what you are doing to help them. A simple, straightforward, reassuring approach is best.

It is Fire Prevention Week, and your crew is at an elementary school teaching fire prevention and timing fire drills. While you are with the second-grade class, a teacher's aide comes running up to your engine saying that there is a child in the kindergarten class having difficulty breathing. You grab your jump bag and follow her to a five-year-old female sitting at her desk in a tripod position, eyes wide with fear, wheezing audibly. Lateesha is her name. Her respirations are rapid and labored, and her skin appears to be pale and grayish. Her teacher tells you that her pediatrician suspects she may be developing asthma.

15. Lateesha's initial vital signs are as follows: respirations 36, pulse 146, BP 120/86. Are they low, normal, or high for a five-year-old? If they are low or high, what would be normal?

16. List five questions you would like to ask Lateesha. Be sure to state them in a manner appropriate for a five-year-old.

    a.

b.

c.

d.

e.

17. The paramedics have arrived, and you must give them a hand-off report. Write 1–8 to show the correct order in which the information should be reported.

    _______ **a.** Lateesha is currently undergoing tests to determine if she has asthma.

    _______ **b.** This is Lateesha. She is five years old. About 20 minutes ago, she became acutely short of breath.

    _______ **c.** Lateesha's medical card states that she takes no medications and has no drug, food, or other types of allergies.

    _______ **d.** We initially found Lateesha sitting in this chair in a tripod position, stating that she was having difficulty breathing, with labored respirations of 36, a pulse of 146, and a BP of 120/86.

    _______ **e.** Lateesha was using some accessory muscles to breathe. She had audible wheezes and was able to talk in only two- or three-word sentences.

    _______ **f.** We applied high-flow oxygen by nonrebreather mask. After a few minutes, it appeared that Lateesha experienced some relief. However, she remains quite short of breath.

    _______ **g.** Lateesha's mother has been called, and she should be here any minute.

    _______ **h.** Lateesha said she became short of breath while playing on the playground.

Lifting and Moving Patients

KEY IDEAS

This chapter provides an overview of how to lift and move patients and equipment safely, without injury to the patients and without injury to you. Key ideas include the following:

◆ Incorrect lifting and handling of patients can worsen their injuries and cause career-ending injuries to rescuers.

◆ There may be instances in which you must move a patient prior to treating him or her due to hazards, inaccessibility, or other problems.

◆ Emergency techniques for moving patients include the shirt drag, blanket drag, and shoulder or forearm drag.

◆ Non-emergency, or non-urgent, moves include the direct ground lift and extremity lift.

◆ Equipment that First Responders should be acquainted with and know how to use properly include standard stretchers, the stair chair, and backboards.

1. List four basic safety rules of lifting any object.

   a.

   b.

   c.

   d.

2. The key to preventing injury during lifting, carrying, moving, reaching, pushing, and pulling is:
   a. correct alignment of your spine.
   b. balance, strength, and attitude.
   c. to keep your knees slightly bent.
   d. to lock your elbows, wrists, and knees.

3. In a power lift, you should _______ to splint your vulnerable lower back area.
   a. avoid excessive slouch or swayback
   b. take a long, deep breath and hold it
   c. relax the muscles of your legs and buttocks
   d. tighten the muscles of your back and abdomen

4. Which one of the following describes good posture while standing?
   a. Knees are locked and pelvis is tucked back.
   b. Chin points out and shoulders are rolled forward.
   c. Chin, sternum, and knees are in vertical alignment.
   d. Ears, shoulders, and hips are in vertical alignment.

5. Which one of the following describes good posture while sitting?
   a. Knees are locked and pelvis is tucked back.
   b. Chin points out and shoulders are rolled forward.
   c. Chin, sternum, and knees are in vertical alignment.
   d. Ears, shoulders, and hips are in vertical alignment.

6. List five conditions under which you would consider making an emergency move of your patient.

   a.

   b.

   c.

   d.

   e.

7. The greatest danger to the patient during an emergency move is the possibility of making a spine injury worse.

_______ True

_______ False

8. Below are the steps a rescuer must take to perform a "forearm drag." Number the following steps 1–5 to show the order in which they should be performed.

_______ Drag the patient toward you.

_______ Stand at the patient's head.

_______ Grasp the patient's forearms.

_______ Slip your hands under the patient's armpits.

_______ Support the patient's head on your own forearms.

9. Rescuers should use an "extremity lift" when the patient has injuries to his or her arms or legs.

_______ True

_______ False

Questions 10, 11, and 12 may have more than one correct answer. Circle the letters next to all statements that seem correct for each question.

10. Portable stretchers are usually used when there:
    a. are multiple patients.
    b. are flights of stairs to navigate.
    c. is not enough space for a standard stretcher.
    d. is a spinal injury accompanied by unresponsiveness.

11. What type of stretcher can be used to lift a patient from a confined area where a larger stretcher will not fit?
    a. stair chair
    b. scoop stretcher
    c. standard stretcher with wheeled legs
    d. vest-type immobilization device

12. Which of the following pieces of equipment should be used for moving a patient with a possible spinal injury?
    a. backboard
    b. stair chair
    c. pole stretcher
    d. blanket stretcher

Read the scenario and answer the questions that follow. Focus on when you may need to move patients.

Your crew is staged at the local high school during the homecoming game. There is to be a big bonfire afterward, and you are there to keep it from spreading or doing any damage. The game is almost over when you hear the spectators start screaming. A section of the old bleachers has collapsed, trapping five people.

13. What are your first responsibilities? Name at least two.

14. Along with school authorities, you are able to move the crowd of spectators away from the collapsed structure, leaving only those trapped at the scene. What would you need to consider in order to make an emergency move of these patients?

15. Decide if you would move each patient described below right away. Write the reason for your answer.

    a. Patient #1 is sitting at the edge of the collapsed structure with a board over her legs. She is complaining only of knee pain and reports that she fell straight down about two feet onto her buttocks.

    b. Patients #2 and #3 are on top of patient #4. Patients #2 and #3 are awake and complaining of leg and arm pain. They are scared because they cannot wake up patient #4 and cannot feel him breathing.

    c. Patient #5 is trapped in some metal debris. He says that he cannot move his legs and that his neck hurts. There are no other dangers around him.

Multiple-Casualty Incidents and Incident Management

This chapter provides an overview of ways in which EMS systems respond to multiple-casualty incidents and your role as a First Responder. Key ideas include the following:

◆ The National Fire Service Incident Management System (IMS) provides a command structure through which to manage multiple-casualty incidents.

◆ EMS sector functions in a multiple-casualty incident include staging, supply, extrication, triage, treatment, transportation, and rehab.

◆ As a fire service First Responder, you will probably be assigned to a role involving patient assessment and treatment.

◆ Triage is a process of classifying sick and injured patients. It is used to determine the order in which each patient receives medical care and transport.

◆ Multiple-casualty incidents can have a severe psychological impact on both patients and rescuers. Strategies for managing these impacts increase the effectiveness of rescuers and help to lessen the long-term problems associated with critical incident stress.

1. IMS has five major functional areas. List them and then give a brief description of each one.

a.

b.

c.

d.

e.

2. *ON SCENE* ◆ At 2:00 A.M. Friday night, two cars are involved in a high-speed, head-on vehicle collision. You are the first on scene. Your first action should be to:
a. perform triage and provide treatment.
b. size up the scene and establish command.
c. block off the roadway and set out flares.
d. request additional resources and personnel.

3. While performing a scene size-up of a multiple-casualty incident, what should you assess for?

a.

b.

c.

d.

e.

f.

g.

4. Use a four-level system to triage the following patients. Write "Priority 1," "Priority 2," "Priority 3," or "Priority 4" in the spaces provided.

_______________ **a.** A patient with shortness of breath and cyanosis

_______________ **b.** A patient with a painful, swollen ankle

_______________ **c.** A patient with an open, deformed injury to the right femur

_______________ **d.** A patient with swelling and deformity to both arms

_______________ **e.** A patient who is unresponsive with no signs of trauma

_______________ **f.** A patient with superficial burns to a forearm

_______________ **g.** A patient with uncontrolled bleeding from a wrist

_______________ **h.** A patient with partial-thickness burns to the hands and feet

_______________ **i.** A patient with controlled bleeding for a laceration to the calf

_______________ **j.** A patient with inhalation burns

_______________ **k.** A patient with abrasions and bruising to the torso

_______________ **l.** A trauma patient with an altered mental status, rapid pulse, and cool, moist skin that is gray looking

_______________ **m.** A patient who has been unresponsive for 20 minutes

5. **ON SCENE** ◆ You are assigned to triage patients involved in a building collapse. Your initial assessment of the following patients is as follows.

Patient 1: Your patient is unresponsive, breathing, and has severe, uncontrolled bleeding to the left lower leg. Your next step should be to:
a. move on to the next patient.
b. use an arterial pressure point.
c. apply high-concentration oxygen.
d. apply a pressure dressing to the wound.

Patient 2: You determine that your patient is not breathing. Your next step should be to:
a. assess for a pulse.
b. move on to the next patient.
c. apply high-concentration oxygen.
d. open the airway with a manual maneuver.

Patient 3: Your patient is unresponsive and breathing. Your next step should be to:
a. assess for a pulse.
b. move on to the next patient.
c. apply high-concentration oxygen.
d. determine if the patient is responsive to pain.

Read the scenario and answer the questions that follow. Remember, establishing an organized approach that correctly sets priorities is the most important determinant of a successful MCI.

You respond along with two other First Responders in a rescue vehicle to a reported head-on collision on the nearby interstate. Your communications center advises you that the closest law enforcement and ambulance responses are approximately 15 and 20 minutes away, respectively. You arrive on scene to find all lanes of the interstate blocked by the collision. It appears that a bread truck crossed the center median and collided head-on with a station wagon carrying six occupants. There is massive damage to both vehicles. Bystanders have set out flares. As the senior member of the rescue crew, you are the initial incident commander.

6. What initial information should you gather during your scene size-up? List a series of questions you would ask when gathering this information.

7. You have identified seven patients, six in the station wagon and one in the bread truck. Use a four-level system to triage them. Write "Priority 1," "Priority 2," "Priority 3," or "Priority 4" in the space provided.

   ___________________ a. An unrestrained 18-month-old female who appears to be unresponsive after being thrown against the windshield of the station wagon. She presents with head and chest injuries, rapid breathing, and a faint brachial pulse.

   ___________________ b. A 37-year-old male, driver of the station wagon. Presents with an altered mental status, from repeating himself to being confused about what has happened. He is pinned by the steering column and has obvious chest injuries and leg fractures.

   ___________________ c. A 38-year-old male, the restrained driver of the bread truck. He presents as alert with significant facial lacerations and neck pain.

   ___________________ d. A 34-year-old female, restrained front-seat passenger of the station wagon. She took the brunt of the bread truck's impact. She appears to be breathless and pulseless with massive head, chest, and pelvic trauma.

                                        e. A 14-year-old male, backseat unrestrained passenger in the station wagon. He has painful, swollen, deformed injuries to both thighs. He also has closed abdominal injuries. He is responsive and screaming.

                                          f. A 9-year-old female, unrestrained back-seat passenger in the station wagon. She was ejected from the car on impact, and was found supine on the median with massive open head injuries and a grossly angulated neck. She is unresponsive and breathing three to four times per minute.

                                          g. A 12-year-old male, restrained back-seat passenger of the station wagon. He has severe abdominal and chest pain and painful, deformed forearms. He presents as alert and crying.

8. Unfortunately, there is no helicopter service available. Bearing in mind that optimally one ambulance should transport only one critical patient, how many ambulances should you request for this incident? Explain your answer.

EMS Operations

KEY IDEAS

This chapter provides a brief overview of some of the operational aspects of out-of-hospital emergency care, including the six basic phases of an emergency response and emergency vehicle safety. Key ideas include the following:

♦ First Responders should have on hand equipment for airway and breathing management, bleeding control and bandaging, and patient assessment. Also, personal protective equipment is necessary.

♦ There are six general phases of an EMS response: preparation, dispatch, en route to the scene, arrival on scene, transfer of care, and post-run activities.

♦ Many First Responders spend a lot of time in traffic, both in cars and on foot at the emergency scene. A safety course and refresher courses are recommended.

♦ Driver safety depends in large part on common sense and good judgment.

♦ First Responders must never compromise their own safety.

♦ Once inside an ambulance compartment, First Responders must protect themselves. The techniques of hanging on and bracing allow for safer movement in the compartment. Securing the patient correctly can protect both the patient and rescuer.

1. Which phase is the formal beginning of an EMS response?
   a. dispatch
   b. preparation
   c. post-run duties
   d. arrival on scene
   e. transfer of care
   f. en route to the scene

2. The emergency medical dispatcher may give specific, life-saving instructions to the caller to perform during which phase of an emergency response?
   a. dispatch
   b. preparation
   c. post-run duties
   d. arrival on scene
   e. transfer of care
   f. en route to the scene

3. While you are en route to the scene of an emergency, you must do which three of the following?
   a. Know the exact location of the emergency.
   b. Report the number of patients and severity of injuries.
   c. Ignore the speed limits, stop signs, and yields.
   d. Notify dispatch when you begin your response.
   e. Wear seat belts at all times.

4. List four basic ways you can improve driving safety on the way to an emergency scene.

   a.

   b.

   c.

   d.

5. As you approach an emergency scene, disengage your seat belt so you can slip out of the vehicle quickly.

   _______ True

   _______ False

6. Once you turn off your lights and siren, you are no longer driving an "authorized" emergency vehicle and you are subject to the laws meant to govern regular traffic.

_______ True

_______ False

7. There are three precautions you can take to protect your hearing while riding in an emergency vehicle. List them.

   a.

   b.

   c.

8. Park alongside the crash scene to protect injured patients from oncoming traffic.

_______ True

_______ False

9. *ON SCENE* ◆ It is midnight and Anthony is at the scene of an emergency that involved falling debris. There are multiple patients, and at first glance some of them look critical. As Anthony enters the scene, he puts on his protective gloves and takes other necessary BSI precautions. He is already wearing his jumpsuit and heavy-duty work boots. What other protective gear, if any, should he be wearing?

◆ ON SCENE: Scene Safety

Read the scenario and answer the questions that follow. Focus on scene safety.

Rescue 723 is dispatched to a motor-vehicle collision. The dispatcher informs the rescuers that there are three patients in one vehicle who are believed to have critical injuries related to the head and chest. The scene is located at First and Division Streets in the village.

10. List at least five safety tips involved in the emergency vehicle response to the scene.

a.

b.

c.

d.

e.

11. Once on scene, you note that police have not yet arrived to control traffic. If you were to perform that task, what would three of your goals be for rerouting traffic?

a.

b.

c.

12. Describe how you would place cones or flares to redirect traffic.

Hazardous Materials

KEY IDEAS

This chapter focuses on how to recognize hazardous materials at the scene of an emergency and how to respond to this threat. Key ideas include the following:

◆ Hazardous materials are substances that pose a threat or unreasonable risk to health, life, or property if they are not properly controlled during manufacture, storage, transportation, use, or disposal.

◆ With billions tons of hazardous materials manufactured annually, hazardous materials accidents caused by equipment failure, vehicle collisions, environmental conditions, or human error are inevitable.

◆ First Responder responsibilities in a hazmat emergency may include identifying the hazmat incident, establishing command and control zones, identifying the substance, and establishing a medical treatment sector.

◆ First Responders must never compromise their own safety when helping to manage a hazardous materials incident.

1. A First Responder's specific responsibilities at a hazmat incident are:

   a.

   b.

   c.

   d.

2. When arriving at the scene of a potential hazmat emergency, the first step is to:
   a. assess the situation from a safe command position.
   b. set up a triage area for potential victims.
   c. begin evacuation from the hot zone.
   d. call for additional resources depending on the nature of the hazmat emergency.

3. Write three possible visual clues to the presence of a hazardous material:

   a.

   b.

   c.

4. When you are called to a possible hazmat emergency, you should station yourself ______ and ______ of the scene.
   a. downhill, downwind
   b. uphill, downwind
   c. uphill, upwind
   d. downhill, upwind

5. Once you have stationed yourself, it is best to look at the possible hazmat scene through your:
   a. binoculars.
   b. closed window.
   c. face mask with HEPA filter.
   d. chemical-resistant jumpsuit.

6. When you report your position and the situation to dispatch, your report should include:

   a.

   b.

   c.

   d.

   e.

   f.

7. The area immediately outside the location of actual contamination is called the:
   a. hot zone.
   b. warm zone.
   c. cold zone.
   d. outer perimeter.

8. The location for all rescuers and equipment not immediately managing the hazmat emergency is known as the:
   a. hot zone.
   b. warm zone.
   c. cold zone.
   d. outer perimeter.

9. *ON SCENE* ◆ You and your partner have arrived at the scene of a hazardous materials incident. A tractor-trailer jack-knifed on the highway, spilling its liquid contents all over the roadway. After sizing up the scene from a distance, you are able to identify the substance as a strong acid. You can see that the driver is still sitting in the cab. He appears badly injured. Acid is bubbling forth from a large gash in the side of the tank. The hazmat team should be at the scene in 10 to 15 minutes. What actions do you wish to take prior to their arrival?

Read the scenario and answer the questions that follow. Always remember to ensure your own safety above all other considerations.

Your crew has responded to a possible inhalation emergency at one of the local vegetable packing plants. The dispatch originally indicated that one patient may have been exposed, and they have dispatched an ambulance from a neighbor company. You arrive to find a chaotic scene. Workers are streaming out of one packing shed, while supervisors are running around, shouting instructions to one another. You find a group of about 20 workers just outside the shed, complaining of headache, dizziness, and some difficulty breathing. The ambulance is still about 10 minutes away.

"What's going on?" you ask one of the workers.

"I think there's bad air in this packing shed," she says.

"What kind of bad air?"

"Who knows? They use different types of gases at this plant."

"Was anyone contaminated by any type of liquid?"

"No, just something in the air."

10. Your first action at this point should be to:
    a. begin initial assessments of the workers.
    b. move the people away from the danger.
    c. go into the building to see if there are more patients.
    d. attempt to identify the gas causing the incident.

11. A supervisor tells you that he is pretty sure the gas in the packing shed is carbon monoxide. Based on this information, is it really necessary to establish hot, warm, and cold zones, or to have a hazmat team dispatched? Explain.

12. A packing plant supervisor tells you that the contaminated shed has been evacuated except for three workers who cannot be accounted for. Hazmat personnel are still five to seven minutes away from the incident. The supervisor and some of the workers want to reenter the shed to look for the missing workers. Do you let them in or do you deny access until the hazmat team arrives?

Fireground Rehabilitation

This chapter provides an overview of emergency incident rehabilitation (EIR). Key ideas include the following:

◆ Stress- and heat-related emergencies are the main causes of on-duty firefighter deaths. Emergency incident rehabilitation (EIR) helps to assure the well-being of personnel who are fighting a fire for a long stretch of time.

◆ As a First Responder, you may be called upon to staff the rehab sector/group. Your role will be to provide a safe area, identify rescuers at risk, medically monitor crews, assure accountability, and update incident command.

CONTENT REVIEW

1. The physical stress of fire fighting can result in cardiac emergencies and sudden death.

    _______ True

    _______ False

2. **ON SCENE** ◆ Firefighters are dealing with a structure fire in a newspaper warehouse. After break, a company officer sees that one crew member, Bill, is suffering from heat exhaustion. He sends Bill to rehab and Bill's other crew members back to fighting the fire. Was the company officer's decision correct? Explain your answer.

3. From the list below, identify the criteria for the proper location of an EIR area.
   a. downwind of the hot zone
   b. out of view of the work area
   c. near running, drinkable water
   d. in a shady, cool area in hot weather
   e. as far away from the staging area as possible

4. The term "accountability" refers to:
   a. needing more than one rehab sector/group at a work site.
   b. evaluating crew members for stress- and heat-related illnesses.
   c. the minimum training required for staffing a rehab sector/group.
   d. tracking rescuers to avoid delay in noticing that one is missing.

5. An ideal layout for a rehab sector/group is to have a separate entry point and a separate exit point.

______ True

______ False

6. Crew members who have a pulse rate greater than _____ per minute at entry are assigned to the medical evaluation/treatment area.
   a. 120
   b. 100
   c. 80
   d. 60

7. As a rule, rescuers sent to the rehab sector/group should remain there a minimum of _____ minutes.
   a. 80
   b. 60
   c. 40
   d. 20

ON SCENE: A Structure Fire

Read the scenario and answer the questions that follow. Focus on your role as an EMS First Responder.

Your engine company has been assigned to establish a rehab sector/group at the site of a three-alarm warehouse fire. You are assigned to assist with the medical evaluations of firefighters.

8. What are four functions you may be required to carry out?

   a.

   b.

c.

d.

9. What are three standard criteria that would require firefighters to report to rehab?

   a.

   b.

   c.

10. List at least eight signs and symptoms of potential life threats related to stress- and heat-related illnesses.

    a.

    b.

    c.

    d.

    e.

    f.

    g.

    h.

CHAPTER 26

EMS Rescue Operations

KEY IDEAS

This chapter provides an overview of rescue operations at motor-vehicle collision scenes and water-related emergencies. Key ideas include the following:

◆ Safety is always your top priority. Never attempt vehicle stabilization and patient extrication or a water rescue unless you have been specifically trained to do so, you are properly equipped, and you have assistance from other trained rescuers.

◆ The most important initial action when faced with an extrication problem is to size up the scene, determining the number of patients, the presence of any scene hazards, and whether or not you have the proper resources.

◆ Suspect any vehicle of being unstable until it is made stable.

◆ Doors and windows provide simple access to patients. If complex access is required, call for rescuers who have the training and equipment.

◆ In vehicle-collision emergencies, spinal precautions should be taken on all patients prior to extrication. In water emergencies, patients with suspected spine injuries should have their spines stabilized while still in the water.

1. **ON SCENE** ◆ As you drive to work, you witness a pickup truck slam into a telephone pole. The single occupant, a male in his 30s, appears to be awake but dazed. The windshield of the truck is starred, and the steering column is bent. There appears to be no fire danger. You radio in for police and a fire and ambulance response. Meanwhile, what steps should you take to manage the scene and the patient?

2. Identify the statements below that are true about setting flares at the scene of a vehicle collision.
   a. Flares should be set 10–15 feet (3–5 m) apart.
   b. The flare string should extend 100 feet (30 m) toward traffic.
   c. The danger zone is a 50-foot (15 m) radius around the wrecked cars.
   d. If the road has two lanes, position flares in the nearest lane only.
   e. Extend the flare string if heavy trucks travel the road.

3. Complex access is access by which no tools are needed. Simple access is access that requires tools and specialized equipment.

   _______ True

   _______ False

4. **ON SCENE** ◆ You are at the scene of an "auto vs. tree" and find the vehicle with massive front and side damage. The patient inside appears to be unconscious with labored respirations. Provided the vehicle is properly stabilized, the two best methods for accessing this patient would be to:
   a. remove the windshield.
   b. break a side or rear window.
   c. attempt entry through a door.
   d. cut through the top of the car.

5. If you must break a window to gain access to a patient trapped in a crashed vehicle, break the window farthest from your patient.

   _______ True

   _______ False

6. There is a significant difference between warm- and cold-water drownings. Describe what that difference is.

7. Never try a water rescue unless you meet all of the four basic criteria for doing so. List them.

a.

b.

c.

d.

8. *ON SCENE* ◆ You are enjoying a sunny afternoon at a lake when you hear that a swimmer is in trouble just offshore. You run over to the place where a group of people has gathered and spot a woman in her 20s thrashing about in the water about 100 feet (30 m) offshore. Witnesses tell you that she was floating on an inflatable raft that lost air and sank. Briefly describe three techniques that might be used to rescue her.

a.

b.

c.

Read the scenario and answer the questions that follow. Remember that effective resuscitation of a patient depends on an accurate assessment and aggressive treatment of the patient's airway, breathing, and circulation.

You have just finished lunch at the fire station when one of the calls you dread the most is dispatched: "Child in the water, possible drowning." As you respond to a nearby resort, your dispatcher updates you, stating that lifeguards have located an unresponsive five-year-old in the lake. A paramedic ambulance is approximately 10 minutes behind you.

9. What sort of management planning could you complete with your two fellow crew members en route to this call? How might you divide the workload for this call among the three of you?

Your patient has a radial pulse of 50. You have cleared her airway and have taken over rescue breathing via bag-valve-mask supplied with 100% oxygen. You decided to use a jaw-thrust maneuver to open her airway, and you inserted an oropharyngeal airway. Despite several attempts, you are not able to achieve adequate ventilations. Your patient has minimal chest rise with ventilation. You are somewhat concerned that she may have some sort of spinal injury, but you find yourself becoming more concerned with the lack of chest rise with ventilations.

10. Describe at three methods you would use to open her airway and achieve adequate ventilations.

11. One of her parents approaches you and asks, "How is Maggie doing? Is she going to be all right?" At this point, Maggie's heart rate is 50 beats per minute. She is unresponsive and still breathless. The paramedics are about one minute away. Write out a short response to this parent.

12. The paramedics have just shown up. Number the following sentences 1–7 in order to develop a coherent, efficient report.

_______ **a.** Maggie remains unresponsive. She is not breathing on her own but does have a strong radial pulse of 88.

_______ **b.** When we arrived, Maggie was unresponsive, with a slow radial pulse.

_______ **c.** Maggie is an unresponsive, near-drowning victim. She was submerged for about three to four minutes.

_______ **d.** The lifeguards spotted her about 20 feet offshore in about three feet of water. They rescued her and began rescue breathing immediately.

_______ **e.** We suctioned her airway, inserted an oropharyngeal airway, and began ventilating with 100% oxygen via BVM.

_______ **f.** We do not find any associated trauma.

_______ **g.** Maggie has no medical history, takes no medications, and has no medication allergies.

Appendix

Fire Service First Responder Skill Summary Sheets

Manual Stabilization of Cervical Spine — 160

Airway Assessment — 161

The Oropharyngeal Airway — 162

The Nasopharyngeal Airway — 163

Oxygen Administration — 164

One-Rescuer Adult CPR — 165

Two-Rescuer Adult CPR — 166

External Bleeding Control — 167

Shock Management — 168

Splinting — 169

Sling and Swathe — 170

Fire Service First Responder
Skill Summary Sheets

MANUAL STABILIZATION OF CERVICAL SPINE

Skill Summary	Check If Performed
1 Place your hands on both sides of the patient's head.	
2 Hold the head firmly and steadily in a neutral, in-line position.	
3 Maintain manual stabilization until the patient is completely immobilized.	
Note: If the patient's head is not already in a neutral, in-line position when you begin, gently guide it there. If there is any pain or if you feel resistance, stop immediately and stabilize the head in the position in which it was found.	

Name ____ Date __________

AIRWAY ASSESSMENT

Skill Summary	Check If Performed
1 Open the airway. —Use a jaw-thrust maneuver for a trauma patient. —Use a head-tilt/chin-lift for a medical patient.	
2 Inspect the airway. —For a responsive patient, listen to him speak and answer questions. —For an unresponsive patient, open the mouth with a cross-finger technique.	
3 Clear the airway if necessary.	
4 Assess breathing, determining presence and adequacy.	
Note: If the patient is breathless or breathing is inadequate, provide ventilatory support.	

Fire Service First Responder
Skill Summary Sheets

THE OROPHARYNGEAL AIRWAY

Skill Summary	Check If Performed
1 Select the proper size airway.	
2 Open the patient's mouth. If necessary, use the cross-finger technique.	
3 In an adult, insert the airway upside down, with the top pointing toward the roof of the patient's mouth.	
4 Advance the airway gently until you meet resistance.	
5 Rotate the airway 180° clockwise while you continue to advance it, until the flange rests on the patient's front teeth.	

Note: In an infant or child, use a tongue depressor and insert the airway in its normal upright position. Do not rotate it.

Fire Service First Responder
Skill Summary Sheets

THE NASOPHARYNGEAL AIRWAY

Skill Summary	Check If Performed
1 Select the proper size airway.	
2 Lubricate the device with a sterile, water-soluble lubricant.	
3 Insert the airway posteriorly, with the beveled end toward the septum when it is inserted in the right nostril.	
4 Advance the airway gently and close to the midline along the floor of the nostril and straight back into the nasopharynx.	
Note: If the airway cannot be inserted in one nostril, try the other nostril.	

**Fire Service First Responder
Skill Summary Sheets**

OXYGEN ADMINISTRATION

Skill Summary	Check If Performed
1 Identify the cylinder as oxygen, and remove the protective seal from the tank.	
2 Crack the main cylinder for one second to remove dust and debris.	
3 Place the yoke of the regulator over the cylinder valve and align the pins.	
4 Hand-tighten the T-screw on the regulator.	
5 Open the main cylinder valve to check the pressure.	
6 Attach the proper delivery device (nonrebreather mask or nasal cannula) to the regulator.	
7 Adjust the flow meter to the appropriate liter flow (nonrebreather mask—10–15 liters per minute; nasal cannula—no more than 6 liters per minute).	
8 Apply the oxygen delivery device to the patient.	

Note: When you are ready to discontinue oxygen administration, remove the device from the patient. Then shut off the control valve until liter flow is at zero. Shut off the main cylinder valve. Then bleed the valves by leaving the control valve open until the needle or ball indicator returns to zero.

**Fire Service First Responder
Skill Summary Sheets**

ONE-RESCUER ADULT CPR

Skill Summary	Check If Performed
1 Determine unresponsiveness.	
2 Open the airway, and assess breathing.	
3 If no breathing, provide two slow breaths (1.5 to 2 seconds each). Watch for chest rise, and allow for exhalation between breaths.	
4 Feel for a carotid pulse.	
5 If no pulse, provide cycles of 15:2 compressions and ventilations at a rate of 80–100 compressions per minute.	
6 After four cycles (about one minute), assess pulse.	
7 If there is no pulse, repeat steps 5 through 6.	

Fire Service First Responder
Skill Summary Sheets

TWO-RESCUER ADULT CPR

Skill Summary	Check If Performed
1 Determine unresponsiveness.	
2 Open the airway, and assess breathing.	
3 If no breathing, Rescuer #1 should provide two slow breaths (1.5 to 2 seconds each). Watch for chest rise, and allow for exhalation between breaths.	
4 Rescuer #1 should feel for a carotid pulse.	
5 If no pulse, Rescuer #2 should provide 5 compressions at a rate of 80–100 per minute. Rescuer #1 should provide one slow breath after each 5 compressions. Continue 5:1 cycle for one minute.	
6 Rescuer #1 should assess pulse.	
7 If there is no pulse, repeat steps 5 through 6.	

Fire Service First Responder
Skill Summary Sheets

EXTERNAL BLEEDING CONTROL

Skill Summary	Check If Performed
1 Apply direct pressure to the wound with a gloved hand or sterile dressing.	
2 Elevate the bleeding extremity.	
3 If bleeding is not controlled, use the appropriate pressure point.	
4 Once bleeding is controlled in an extremity, immobilize the limb by splinting.	

**Fire Service First Responder
Skill Summary Sheets**

SHOCK MANAGEMENT

Skill Summary	Check If Performed
1 Maintain an open airway and adequate breathing.	
2 Prevent any further blood loss.	
3 Position the patient properly.	
4 Keep the patient warm, but avoid overheating.	
5 Provide care for specific injuries while waiting for EMS crews to arrive.	
Note: Comfort, calm, and reassure the patient, and be sure to withhold all food and drink.	

**Fire Service First Responder
Skill Summary Sheets**

SPLINTING

Skill Summary	Check If Performed
1 Stabilize the limb, and assess pulse, movement, and sensation below the injury site.	
2 Cut away clothing to expose the injury.	
3 Control bleeding, if any, and dress and bandage the wound.	
4 Pad the splint.	
5 Secure the limb to the splint, and reassess pulse, movement, and sensation below the injury site.	

Name ____   **Date** _____________

**Fire Service First Responder
Skill Summary Sheets**

SLING AND SWATHE

Skill Summary	Check If Performed
1 Place a pad between the arm and chest.	
2 Support the injured arm with a sling.	
3 Immobilize the arm with a swathe.	

Chapter 1: Introduction to the EMS System

1. **a** *(p. 3)*
2. Answers may include the following: *(p. 5)*
   a. *Regulation and policy*—Each state must have laws, regulations, policies, and procedures that govern its EMS system. It also is required to provide leadership to local jurisdictions.
   b. *Resources management*—Each state must have central control of EMS resources so all patients have equal access to acceptable emergency care.
   c. *Human resources and training*—Ambulance staff must be trained to at least the EMT-Basic level.
   d. *Transportation*—Patients must be safely and reliably transported by ground or air ambulance.
   e. *Facilities*—Every seriously ill or injured patient must be delivered in a timely manner to an appropriate medical facility.
   f. *Communications*—A system for public access to the EMS system must be in place. Communication among dispatcher, fire service personnel, other EMS providers, and medical facilities also must be possible.
   g. *Public information and education*—EMS personnel should participate in programs designed to educate the public. The programs are to focus on the prevention of injuries and how to properly access the EMS system.
   h. *Medical oversight*—Each EMS system must have a physician as a medical director.
   i. *Trauma systems*—Each state must develop a system of specialized care for trauma patients, including one or more trauma centers and rehabilitation programs. It must also develop systems for assigning and transporting patients to those facilities.
   j. *Evaluation*—Each state must have a quality improvement system in place for continuing evaluation and upgrading of the state's EMS system.
3. True. *(p. 5)*
4. The four levels of out-of-hospital care providers are First Responder, EMT-Basic, EMT-Intermediate, and EMT-Paramedic. *(p. 6)*
5. In your role as a First Responder, you must: *(pp. 8-9)*
   a. Protect your safety and the safety of your crew, the patient, and bystanders.
   b. Gain access to the patient.
   c. Assess the patient in order to identify life-threatening problems.
   d. Alert additional EMS resources, when needed.
   e. Provide emergency medical care to the patient based on assessment findings.
   f. Assist other EMS personnel when requested.
   g. Participate in record keeping and data collection as required.
   h. Act as liaison with other public safety workers.
6. True. *(p. 10)*

7. a. Direct medical control occurs when the medical director or another physician directs an EMS rescuer at the scene of an emergency by way of a telephone, radio, or in person.
   b. Indirect medical control includes such things as system design, quality management, standing orders, and protocols. *(p. 10)*
8. False. *(p. 10)*
9. True. *(p. 10)*
10. Acknowledge the information, but you must assess the patient yourself. *(pp. 8-10)*
11. You must alert additional EMS resources, provide care based on continued assessment, and participate in record keeping as required by your state or agency. Be sure to also maintain a caring attitude. *(pp. 8-10)*
12. Any three: Assist other EMS agencies as requested. Report what you found in your assessment, what you did, and if it worked. Maintain a caring attitude. Maintain a professional appearance and attitude. *(pp. 8-10)*

Chapter 2: Scene Safety and the Well-Being of the First Responder

1. **a–g.** High-stress situations include incidents in which there are multiple casualties or that involve injury to an infant or a child, death of a patient, an amputation, violence, abuse, or injury or death of a coworker. *(p. 17)*
2. **d** *(p. 21)*
3. Certain foods increase the body's response to stress. So you might cut down on sugar and caffeine. (Watch out, soft drinks as well as coffee and tea may have caffeine.) Avoid fatty foods, and eat more low-fat carbohydrates. While at work, eat often but in small amounts. Avoid alcohol and other kinds of self-medication. Exercise regularly, and learn to relax. If at all possible, a First Responder might also request work shifts that allow for more time with family and friends or ask for a rotation of duty to a less stressful assignment. *(pp. 18-19)*
4. **c** *(pp. 19-20)*
5. **a** *(p. 20)*
6. **d** *(p. 20)*
7. You would access CISD if you have been involved in the serious injury or death of a rescuer in the line of duty; a multiple-casualty incident; the suicide of an emergency worker; an event that attracts media attention; the injury or death of someone you know; any disaster; injury or death of an infant or a child. Also access CISD after any event that has unusual impact on you, such as an incident in which injury or death of a civilian was caused by a rescuer, the death of one of your patients occurred, child abuse or neglect was suspected or confirmed, an event that threatens your life, or an incident that involves distressing sights, sounds, or smells. *(p. 20)*

8. **c** *(p. 23)*
9. **a** *(p. 24)*
10. **d** *(p. 24)*
11. **b** *(p. 25)*
12. **d** *(p. 24)*
13. You should always put on protective gloves before you approach your patient. In addition, the appropriate personal protective equipment for each circumstance described is as follows: *(p. 26)*
    a. protective gloves
    b. eye protection, gloves, gown, mask
    c. protective gloves
    d. protective gloves, plus a pocket face mask with one-way valve to perform artificial ventilation during CPR. Eye protection may also be wise, since patients who are resuscitated may vomit.
    e. protective gloves
14. **a.** No—A downed power line does not need to look "hot" to be a potential source of electrocution. Call for specialists to secure the scene before you enter. *(p. 29)*
    b. No—Crowds of people can be very dangerous, especially when violence has occurred. Call for police assistance. *(p. 29)*
    c. Yes—You may enter a scene the police tell you they have secured. *(p. 29)*
15. You should be concerned about the bloody vomit on his clothing as well as his infected sputum and other fluids related to his respiratory problem. *(pp. 22-27)*
16. Wear gloves, as you always should. Because of the potential for more vomiting, also wear eye protection, a mask, and possibly a gown. *(pp. 22-27)*
17. This First Responder is obviously not being careful about protecting her own well-being. Though she may not be able to contract HIV from touching the patient's vomit, she should know that other contagious diseases can be contracted by doing so. While there may be only a small amount of bloody vomit to avoid, it is always best to go into a scene prepared for the worst. After all, the patient may start vomiting again and more profusely. *(pp. 22-27)*
18. Practice aggressive handwashing with soap and hot water, and change any soiled clothing. This clothing should be bagged and then washed in hot, soapy water for at least 25 minutes. Take a hot shower yourself and rinse thoroughly. *(pp. 22-27)*

Chapter 3: **Legal and Ethical Issues**

1. **b** *(p. 38)*
2. **b** *(p. 39)*
3. **c** *(p. 39)*
4. **a** *(p. 39)*
5. First tell the patient who you are. Identify your level of training, and then carefully explain your plan for emergency care. Make sure you identify both the benefits and the risks. To make sure the patient understands, question him or her briefly. *(p. 39)*
6. **c** *(p. 39)*
7. Provide emergency care as you would for any patient who needs it. In the absence of a valid advance directive, you have no other choice but to assume implied consent. *(pp. 39-41)*
8. **a** *(p. 43)*
9. Try one last time to persuade the patient to accept treatment or transport. Be sure the patient is able to make a rational, informed decision. Consult medical direction as required by local protocol. Have the patient and a witness sign a refusal or "release from liability" form. Encourage the patient to seek help if certain symptoms develop. Advise the patient to call EMS again immediately if he or she has a change of mind. *(pp. 41, 43)*
10. **b** *(p. 43)*
11. **a** *(p. 43)*
12. **c** *(p. 45)*
13. Yes, he is employed as a First Responder, and he is on the job. He must provide the emergency care he's trained and contracted to provide. *(p. 43)*
14. No, he does not have a duty to act. He's not on call and, even if he was, his contract is with his employer, not the general public. *(p. 43)*
15. **c** *(p. 44)*
16. Absolutely. You have no way of knowing if the chest pain is serious or not. A physician needs to examine the patient before such a decision can be made. *(p. 38)*
17. You might explain to Mr. Boyd that he may have had or may be having a heart attack. If so, it is imperative that he be seen immediately to reduce the chance of permanent damage to his heart. Also, if he is having a heart attack, a delay in treatment could be very serious, even fatal. You might also suggest to Mrs. Boyd that she speak to her husband. He may listen to her. *(pp. 41, 43)*
18. You shouldn't. Mr. Boyd has the right to refuse treatment and transport. He is fully alert and in control of his mental faculties. There is no sign of intoxication, no history of mental illness, and he generally appears to be rational. He is allowed to disagree with any medical opinion of his condition. As long as he understands that he may be having a heart attack, as well as the risks involved with delaying treatment, EMS personnel have no recourse. *(pp. 41, 43)*

Chapter 4: **The Human Body**

1. In the anatomical position, a patient's body stands erect with arms down at the sides, palms facing you. In the lateral recumbent position, the patient is lying on his or her left or right side. In the prone position, a patient is lying face down on his or her stomach. In the supine position, a patient is lying face up on his or her back. *(p. 52)*
2. **a** *(p. 52)*
3. **c** *(p. 52)*
4. **d** *(p. 53)*
5. **c** *(p. 52)*
6. **b** *(p. 52)*
7. **a** *(p. 52)*
8. **c** *(p. 53)*
9. **d** *(p. 53)*
10. **a** *(p. 52)*

11.

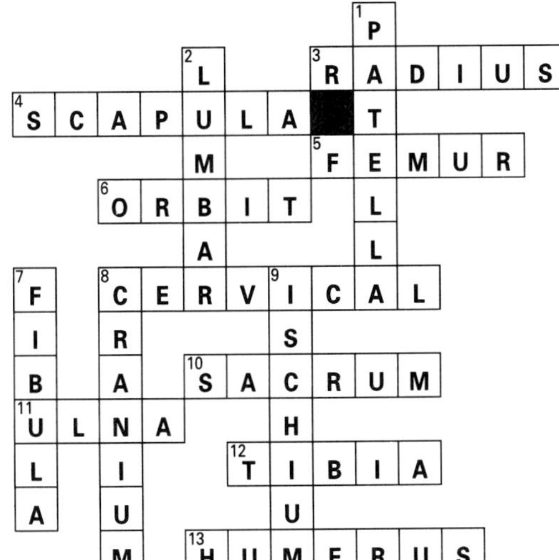

12. **d** *(p. 53)*
13. **c** *(pp. 53, 55)*
14. **d** *(pp. 53, 55)*
15. **a** *(pp. 53, 55)*
16. **c** *(pp. 53, 55)*
17. **a** *(pp. 53, 55)*
18. **a** *(pp. 53, 55)*
19. **a** *(p. 56)*
20. **c** *(p. 56)*
21. **b** *(p. 56)*
22. **c** *(p. 56)*
23. **a** *(p. 56)*
24. Skeletal muscles are voluntary muscles that shape the body, form its walls, and make possible all deliberate acts such as walking and chewing. Smooth muscles are involuntary muscles found in the walls of organs, ducts, and blood vessels. A person has little or no control over smooth muscle. *(pp. 56, 59)*
25. **c** *(p. 59)*
26. **f** *(pp. 59, 61)*
27. **a** *(p. 59)*
28. **a** *(p. 59)*
29. *(p. 61)*
   a. smaller
   b. more
   c. more
   d. more, softer
30. **d** *(p. 61)*
31. The brachial pulse point may be felt in the upper arm; the radial pulse point, at the wrist; the femoral pulse point, in the thigh; and the carotid pulse point, at the neck. *(p. 61)*
32. **b** *(p. 66)*
33. **a** *(pp. 66-67)*
34. **b** *(p. 67)*
35. **d** *(p. 67)*
36. The liver, gallbladder, and colon may be injured. The right kidney is behind these organs, so it is much less likely to be injured from a blow to the anterior thorax. *(pp. 53, 55)*
37. Her confusion may be the result of an injury to the nervous system, specifically her brain. She has a bruised forehead and was not wearing a helmet. Any significant impact to the head can cause a patient's thinking to become confused. *(pp. 61-63)*

38. Treat the breathing problem before the other injuries. A body can survive only a few minutes without oxygen. Any significant injury to this system can cause an immediate threat to life. Scraped skin and abdominal pain can wait. *(p. 59)*
39. The patient appears to have a fractured tibia just distal to the knee, which has caused the lower leg to rotate externally or laterally. *(pp. 52-53)*

Chapter 5: Airway

1. 6, 2, 1, 4, 5, 3 *(pp. 75-76)*
2. a, b, c *(p. 76)*
3. a, b, d *(p. 76)*
4. Adult—12-20 breaths per minute.
Child—15-30 breaths per minute.
Infant—25-50 breaths per minute. *(p. 77)*
5. **b** *(p. 77)*
6. **b** *(p. 77)*
7. **b** *(p. 77)*
8. **c** *(p. 78)*
9. Place the hand closest to the patient's head on the patient's forehead. Apply firm, backward pressure with the palm of your hand to tilt the head back. Place the fingertips of your other hand under the bony part of the lower jaw. Lift the chin forward, and, at the same time, support the jaw and tilt the head back. Continue to press the other hand on the patient's forehead to keep the head tilted back. *(p. 78)*
10. **c** *(p. 78)*
11. **b** *(pp. 78-80)*
12. **d** *(pp. 78-80)*
13. False. Use an oropharyngeal airway if your patient is unresponsive with no gag reflex. *(p. 81)*
14. **d** *(p. 81)*
15. Select the proper size. Open the patient's mouth. Insert the oropharyngeal airway upside down, with the tip pointing toward the roof of the patient's mouth. Advance the adjunct gently until you encounter resistance. Turn the airway 180° until the flat flange at the top rests on the patient's front teeth. *(p. 81)*
16. **c** *(p. 82)*
17. True. *(p. 82)*
18. **c** *(p. 83)*
19. Select the proper size. Lubricate it with a sterile, water soluble lubricant. Insert the airway posteriorly. It is properly in place when the flange lies against the flare of the nostril. *(p. 83)*
20. **d** *(p. 83)*
21. **a** *(p. 83)*
22. **c** *(pp. 83-84)*
23. 1, 4, 5, 3, 2 *(p. 86)*
24. **c** *(p. 86)*
25. Look for the rise and fall of the patient's chest. Listen for air coming out of the patient's mouth and nose. Feel for air coming out of the patient's nose and mouth. *(p. 87)*
26. Inadequate breathing may be characterized by rates less than 8 respirations per minute in an adult, less than 10 in a child, and less than 20 in an infant. *(p. 87)*
27. a, b, c, d, e, f, i, j, k, l, m *(pp. 87-88)*

28. Any four: Rate of respiration is adequate. Force of air is consistent. Force of air is also sufficient to cause the chest to rise during each ventilation. The patient's heart rate decreases or returns to normal. The patient's color improves. *(p. 88)*

29. The chest does not rise and fall with each ventilation. The ventilation rate is too fast or too slow. The patient's heart rate does not decrease or return to normal. *(p. 88)*

30. b, c, d *(p. 88)*

31. True. *(p. 89)*

32. Position the mask, and create a seal. Open the patient's airway, and deliver two slow breaths. Determine if the ventilations are adequate. If successful, continue ventilations at the proper rate. If unsuccessful, reposition the patient's head and try again. If still unsuccessful, treat for a foreign body airway obstruction. *(p. 89)*

33. *Adult*—10-12 breaths per minute at 1.5 to 2.0 seconds each.
Child—20 breaths per minute at 1.0 to 1.5 seconds each.
Infant—20 breaths per minute at 1.0 to 1.5 seconds each.
Newborn—40 breaths per minute at 1.0 to 1.5 seconds each. *(p. 89)*

34. b *(p. 89)*

35. d *(p. 92)*

36. a *(p. 92)*

37. **a.** Be gentle when you open the infant's airway. Position the head carefully. Keep the baby's head in a neutral position. Remember the airway is more flexible than an adult's and can be easily overextended. *(p. 93)*
b. The rescuer may be able to form a seal with his or her mouth over the infant's mouth and nose. If a pocket mask is being used, place it on the infant's face in an upside-down position. *(p. 93)*
c. Deliver 20 breaths per minute, each breath lasting 1 to 1.5 seconds. *(p. 89)*

38. a *(p. 93)*

39. c, d, f, g, h, i *(p. 96)*

40. c *(p. 101)*

41. **a.** Allow the patient to relieve a partial obstruction unaided. Any assistance you give could potentially create a complete obstruction. *(p. 102)*

42. False. Back blows are not recommended for adults. *(p. 102)*

43. **a.** Get in position behind the patient, with your arms around the patient's waist.
b. Position your hands, with thumb side of your fist on the middle of the patient's abdomen.
c. Perform an abdominal thrust.
d. If the first thrust does not dislodge the foreign body, continue until it is expelled or the patient becomes unresponsive. *(pp. 102-104)*

44. d *(pp. 105-106)*

45. e, f, g. According to AHA guidelines, you would manage any child over the age of eight the same way you would manage an adult. *(p. 106)*

46. False. Suspect a foreign body airway obstruction. *(p. 106)*

47. True. *(p. 107)*

48. 2, 5, 4, 3, 1, *(p. 107)*

49. c *(p. 107)*

50. 2, 3, 4, 1, 5, *(p. 108)*

51. Even though you understand how upset the family is, you must place the needs of the patient first. Get control of the scene. Move people out of the way so that you can take care of Gracie. *(p. 77)*

52. No. Your first step is to assess and open Gracie's airway. Before a patient can receive artificial ventilation, he or she must have an open airway. *(p. 89)*

53. **a.** 3, **b.** 1, **c.** 2 *(p. 89)*

54. Reduce the force of your ventilations. Check to be sure the patient's head is in a neutral position. Be sure to allow the patient to exhale fully between ventilations. *(p. 93)*

55. Suction or quickly wipe out Gracie's mouth with gauze pads. Wipe off her face, too, and return to ventilations. *(p. 93)*

56. Always reassess your patient whenever there is a status change.

Chapter 6: Circulation

1. **a.** lungs
   b. sternum
   c. two-sided
   d. left
   e. right
   f. pressure
   g. pulse *(pp. 115-116)*

2. **a.** artery
   b. brachial
   c. carotid
   d. radial *(pp. 115-116)*

3. Early access, early CPR, early defibrillation, early advanced care. *(pp. 116-117)*

4. The rescuer is exhausted and is unable to continue. The patient is turned over to another trained rescuer or to the hospital staff. The patient is resuscitated. The patient has been declared dead by a proper authority. *(p. 117)*

5. d *(p. 117)*

6. Clockwise: heart, xiphoid process, spleen, stomach, liver, sternum, lungs. *(p. 129)*

7. b *(p. 118)*

8. a *(p. 118)*

9. unresponsive, breathless, pulseless *(p. 117)*

10. **a.** 15:2
    b. 15:2
    c. 5:1
    d. 5:1 *(p. 121)*

11. **a.** Two or three fingers on lower half of sternum.
    b. Heel of one hand on lower half of sternum.
    c. Two hands on lower half of sternum.
    d. Two hands on lower half of sternum. *(p. 121)*

12. *(p.121)*

	Infant	Child	Adult
Rate	at least 100 per minute	100 per minute	80 to 100 per minute
Depth	½ to 1 inches (15 to 25 mm)	1 to ½ inches (25 to 40 mm)	1½ to 2 inches (40 to 50 mm)

13. 2, 3, 6, 5, 1, 4, 7 *(pp. 121-122)*
14. Disagree. This student's hand placement could easily result in injuring the patient's liver. His hand placement should be two fingers' distance above the xiphoid process. *(pp. 119-123)*
15. Chest compressions need to be smooth in order to provide the best circulation of blood through the patient's body. Jabbing or jerking movements may cause the blood to spurt from the heart and will not increase blood circulation. *(p. 123)*
16. For one-rescuer CPR, the ratio of compressions to ventilations is 15:2, and you should check the patient's pulse every two to three minutes. For two-rescuer CPR, the ratio of compressions to ventilations is 5:1, and you should check the patient's pulse every two to three minutes. *(pp. 121-122, 125)*
17. CPR may need to be stopped for more than five seconds if the patient is in a position where effective CPR cannot be performed. In this case, the patient must be moved. *(p. 126)*
18. Any three: fracture of the sternum, pneumothorax, hemothorax, cuts and bruises to the lungs, lacerations to the liver. *(p. 128)*
19. c *(p. 128)*
20. d *(p. 128)*
21. False. Attempt to resuscitate an infant for one minute before activating the EMS. *(p. 128)*
22. b *(p. 131)*
23. The crunch may mean the patient's rib cartilage separated. Check your hand placement, but continue with CPR. Remember, the alternative is that the patient dies. *(p. 128)*
24. Your first action should be to introduce yourself to the person who is providing CPR. Tell him you are a First Responder, a trained EMS rescuer. Ask him if he wants you to assist. *(p. 122)*
25. If he wants you to assist, get in position at the patient's head. Then check the patient's pulse while a compression is being performed. When the compression is complete, provide two ventilations and check the patient's pulse. Then, if necessary, you may resume CPR. *(p. 122)*
26. This person needs some coaching. He needs to reposition his hands so that he is compressing the lower half of the patient's sternum, two finger-widths above the xiphoid process. He needs to compress the chest more forcefully—$1\frac{1}{2}$ to 2 inches (40 to 50 mm) in depth. Finally, he needs to compress the patient's chest at a rate of 80 to 100 compressions per minute. *(p. 121)*

Chapter 7: Automated External Defibrillation

1. Defibrillation is the application of an electric shock to the chest of an unresponsive, breathless, pulseless patient. *(p. 139)*
2. a *(p. 139)*
3. Begin CPR. The AED is not used on patients younger than 12 years of age. *(pp. 140-141)*
4. No, because this patient is breathing and has a pulse. The AED is only used on breathless, pulseless patients. *(pp. 140-141)*
5. a. No. Do not use an AED on patients who weigh less than 90 pounds. *(p. 141)*
   b. No. Do not use an AED on patients younger than 12 years of age. *(p. 141)*
   c. Yes. *(p. 141)*
   d. Yes. *(p. 141)*
6. Defibrillation is most likely to be successful when it is attempted as soon as possible. CPR maintains a patient until defibrillation can be attempted. *(p. 141)*
7. c *(p. 143)*
8. 1, 6, 5, 3, 4, 2, 7 *(pp. 143-144)*
9. a *(p. 145)*
10. Remove the patch and wipe off the chest with a towel. *(p. 143)*
11. Make sure no one touches the patient or the AED while the AED is in operation. *(p. 140)*
12. Assist with ventilations. *(p. 144)*
13. a. Place him in a recovery position.
    b. Apply high-concentration oxygen if you are allowed to do so.
    c. Keep the AED attached to the patient, and continue to assess his condition until you transfer care to more highly trained EMS personnel. *(pp. 144-145)*

Chapter 8: Scene Size-up

1. Any two: wear safe clothing, prepare equipment properly, carry a portable radio, plan your safety roles ahead of time. *(pp. 153-154)*
2. a. Any indication that violence has taken or may take place should be considered a sign of potential danger.
   b. When people use alcohol or drugs, their behavior can be unpredictable.
   c. Emergencies are usually very active events. "Absolute silence" is unusual. Anything unusual should be considered a cause for caution. *(p. 154)*
3. Retreat, radio, and reevaluate. *(pp. 154-155)*
4. ill *(p. 155)*
5. injured *(p. 155)*
6. b *(p. 155)*
7. b *(p. 155)*
8. Up-and-over pathways of motion tend to cause major head, neck, chest, and abdominal injuries. Down-and-under pathways of motion tend to yield more injuries to the legs and pelvis. *(pp. 156-157)*
9. *Driver of the sedan:* This patient would probably have few injuries. The combination of safety devices he used are specifically designed to minimize injury resulting from a head-on crash. Aside from some bumps, bruises, strains, and sprains, and possibly a few minor burns from the deployment of the air bag, this patient should be relatively unhurt.
   Driver of the pickup: Expect this patient to have severe injuries. While the lap belt may have kept him from being ejected, this patient could have severe injury to his spine as well as major head, neck, chest, and abdominal injuries. *(pp. 156-159)*
10. a, b, c, d *(pp. 157-158)*
11. c *(p. 157)*
12. d *(pp. 159-160)*

13. **c** *(p. 160)*
14. Yes. While it does not meet the DOT's 15-foot (5 m) requirement for a severe fall, it is close. Plus, the surface the patient landed on is hard, and the patient fell on his chest, which is a region that can incur life-threatening injuries. If you ever have trouble deciding whether or not a mechanism of injury is severe, err on the side of the patient. It is always better to overtreat a patient than to undertreat him. *(p. 160)*
15. False. A low-velocity impact, such as a knife wound, causes injury to the immediate area of impact. A high-velocity injury also affects tissues far from the site of impact. *(p. 161)*
16. False. A high-velocity injury will affect tissues far from the site of impact. *(p. 161)*
17. **c** *(pp. 161, 163)*
18. **a.** rear *(p. 157)*
    b. compression *(p. 156)*
    c. car seat *(p. 159)*
    d. head-on *(pp. 156, 159)*
    e. deceleration *(p. 160)*
    f. ejection *(p. 158)*
    g. side impact *(p. 157)*
    h. sternum *(p. 156)*
    i. blast *(pp. 161, 163)*
    Scrambled letters: aeseltstb
    Unscrambled letters: seat belts
19. Either up-and-over (where the patient's head, chest, and abdomen impact the windshield and steering wheel) or down-and-under (where the patient slips beneath the steering wheel with resulting injuries primarily to the legs and pelvis). *(pp. 156-157)*
20. Probably not. It is doubtful that the air bag would have even deployed, since air bags are designed to deploy in the event of a front-end collision. They generally are not designed to reduce injury from a side impact. *(p. 159)*
21. **a.** Sedan driver—most injured.
    b. Station-wagon driver—likely to have major head, chest, and abdominal injuries.
    c. Compact-car driver—since the concrete barrier did not intrude into the passenger space, and damage to the car was minimal, injuries should only be mild to moderate.
    d. Pickup-truck driver—likeliness of injury is low, plus he had his headrest up. *(pp. 156-159)*
22. **a.** compact car
    b. pickup truck
    c. sedan
    d. station wagon *(pp. 156-159)*

Chapter 9: Patient Assessment

1. Scene size-up, initial assessment, physical exam, patient history, ongoing assessment, patient hand-off. *(p. 168)*
2. **a** *(p. 171)*
3. c, d, f, g, h, i *(pp. 171-177)*
4. 3, 6, 7, 5, 2, 1, 4 *(pp. 171-177)*
5. **c.** This patient needs to be ventilated immediately. Her respirations will not supply her with enough oxygen to survive. *(pp. 171-177)*
6. **a** *(p. 171)*

7. A—The patient is "alert" and oriented to his or her surroundings.
   V—The patient only responds to a "verbal" command.
   P—The patient only responds to "painful" stimuli.
   U—The patient is "unresponsive" or does not respond at all to stimuli. *(pp. 172-173)*
8. verbal *(pp. 172-173)*
9. verbal *(pp. 172-173)*
10. Try to find out from the family if there has been a change. That is, the patient may normally be somewhat confused, but has it worsened with this last episode? *(p. 173)*
11. Expect a responsive child of this age to recognize his or her parents, want to go to them, and probably react negatively to your assessment and treatment. *(p. 173)*
12. **b.** Remember: Airway! Airway! Airway! This patient needs a clear, open airway if she is to survive. Use a jaw-thrust maneuver if the mechanism of injury suggests spine injury. Then clear the airway using suction or a gloved finger. *(pp. 173-174)*
13. Adequate breathing is characterized by adequate rise and fall of the chest, ease of breathing, and adequate respiratory rate. *(p. 174)*
14. **b** *(p. 174)*
15. **b** *(p. 174)*
16. **a** *(p. 175)*
17. **c** *(p. 175)*
18. **d** *(p. 175)*
19. **b** *(p. 176)*
20. Your update report to EMS should include the patient's age and sex, chief complaint, level of responsiveness, plus airway, breathing, and circulation status. *(pp. 176-177)*
21. 6, 3, 1, 5, 4, 2 *(p. 177)*
22. **a.** Yes
    b. No
    c. Yes *(p. 177)*
23. Inspection (looking), auscultation (listening), and palpation (feeling). *(p. 177)*
24. D = deformities, O = open injuries, T = tenderness, S = swelling. *(p. 177)*
25. **a.** The other three injuries can wait. Patients with neck pain require immediate spinal precautions. *(pp. 178-179)*
26. **b** *(pp. 179-180)*
27. **a** *(pp. 181-182)*
28. Respiration, pulse, skin, pupils, and blood pressure. *(p. 182)*
29. True. *(p. 182)*
30. **c** *(p. 182)*
31. **b** *(p. 182)*
32. **d** *(p. 182)*
33. **e** *(p. 182)*
34. **b** *(pp. 182-183)*
35. **b** *(p. 183)*
36. **c** *(p. 183)*
37. **d** *(p. 183)*
38. **b** *(p. 184)*
39. **a.** Cool skin may mean the patient is suffering from shock, heat exhaustion, or exposure to cold.
    b. Hot skin may be the result of fever or heat stroke.

c. Pale skin may be caused by shock, heart attack, fright, faintness, emotional distress, impaired blood flow.

d. Blueness is caused by reduced levels of oxygen as in shock, heart attack, or poisoning.

e. Black-and-blue mottling is the result of blood seeping under the skin, which is usually caused by a blow or severe infection. *(pp. 184-185)*

40. d *(pp. 185-186)*

41. S = signs and symptoms, A = allergies, M = medications, P = pertinent medical history, L = last oral intake, E = events. *(p. 189)*

42. A sign is something that is observable by another person. A symptom cannot be observed by anyone but the patient. So this patient's complaints are symptoms. *(p. 189)*

43. Any question related to signs and symptoms would be appropriate, such as "Describe what you feel" or "Where do you feel the worst?" *(pp. 189-190)*

44. Any question related to allergies would be appropriate, such as "Are you allergic to anything?" "Do you have any allergies to medications?" "Do you have any food allergies or allergies to pollen or dust?" *(p. 190)*

45. Any questions related to medication the patient is currently taking or has recently taken are appropriate. You might ask, for example, "Do you take prescription medication?" or "Have there been any changes in your medications lately?" *(p. 190)*

46. Any question related to the patient's pertinent medical history would be appropriate. For example, you might ask questions such as "Do you see a doctor for anything?" or "Have you ever been admitted to a hospital? For what?" Or you might ask "Have you ever had chest pain before? When? What was done for it?" *(p. 190)*

47. b *(p. 191)*

48. The major elements of the patient hand-off report are: patient age and sex, chief complaint, level of responsiveness, airway status, breathing status, circulation status, physical exam findings, SAMPLE history, and treatment, interventions, and patient's response to them. *(p. 191)*

49. SAMPLE history was omitted. *(p. 191)*

50. a. The ABCs are always first. *(p. 171)*

51. b *(pp. 173-174)*

52. The patient appears to be verbal. *(pp. 172-173)*

53. Immediately reassess the patient's airway, breathing, and circulation. Any time your patient has a dramatic change in level of responsiveness, recheck his or her ABCs.

54. D—Inspect and palpate the skull, face bones, and jaw for signs of deformity, including loose teeth.
O—Inspect for open injuries, especially any injury that bleeds into the airway. Also look in the hair for injuries that may be hidden.
T—Palpating the head for pain or tenderness, even where there is no obvious injury.
S—Inspect injuries to the skull and to facial structures such as areas around the eyes, nose, and mouth for swelling. *(p. 178)*

55. D—Inspect the trachea to see if it is deformed or if it has shifted. Palpate the vertebrae in the posterior (back) of the neck.
O—Inspect for open injuries, and bandage them immediately with an occlusive dressing.
T—Palpate the soft tissues, trachea, and vertebrae for tenderness.
S—Inspect for swelling and listen for a popping or crackling sound under the skin. *(pp. 178-179)*

56. D—Palpate the rib cage for signs of deformity. Do not move the patient in order to examine the back until appropriate spinal precautions have been taken. Palpate the sternum. If the patient is responsive, ask him or her to take a deep breath to determine if it causes pain.
O—Inspect for open injuries. If a wound extends into the chest cavity, bandage it immediately with an occlusive dressing.
T—While palpating the chest, ask the patient if he or she feels any pain to examine for possible internal injuries.
S—Inspect for swelling or any other sign of underlying breathing problems. *(pp. 179-180)*

57. D—Palpate for rigidity or distention.
O—Inspect for open injuries.
T—Palpate each quadrant of the abdomen, but palpate the quadrant where the patient complains of pain last.
S—Inspect for swelling or discoloration of the skin. Check the flanks for pooling of blood. *(p. 180)*

58. D—Palpate for chest wall deformity and for obvious deformity along the length of the spine.
O—Inspect for open injuries, especially for open or sucking chest wounds.
T—Palpate for tenderness.
S—Inspect for swelling and for blood accumulation in the flanks. *(pp. 180-181)*

59. D—Palpate the bones to feel for deformity.
O—Inspect for open injuries.
T—Palpate for tenderness. Palpate with less force if the bones of the pelvis are close to the skin. Palpate with more force if the patient is obese with bones under a considerable amount of tissue. Be sure to palpate the pubis bone.
S—Inspect for swelling and discoloration around the hips. *(p. 181)*

60. D—Inspect and palpate the entire length of each bone and all joints for deformity.
O—Inspect for open injuries.
T—Palpate each extremity for pain and tenderness.
S—Inspect for swelling and discoloration.
Note that any extremity that is painful, swollen, or deformed may be broken and should be manually stabilized until it can be immobilized. You may also wish to check pulses in each extremity, as well as for movement and sensation. *(pp. 181-182)*

Chapter 10: **Cardiac and Respiratory Emergencies**

1. Any five: chest pain or discomfort that may radiate to arms, shoulder, neck, or jaw; difficulty breathing, shortness of breath; unusual pulse; indigestion, nausea, vomiting; sweating; pale, gray, or cyanotic skin; a feeling of impending doom. *(pp. 197-198)*

2. a *(p. 201)*

3. O = onset, P = provocation, Q = quality, R = region, R = radiation, R = relief, S = severity, T = time. *(p. 201)*

4. 5, 3, 2, 1, 4, 6 *(p. 201)*
5. Disagree. This First Responder needs to hit the books. Cardiac emergencies can occur without any chest pain. If signs and symptoms indicate different illnesses or problems, always be prepared to manage the patient as if he or she has the worst one. *(pp. 197-201)*
6. Any seven: inability to speak in full sentences without pausing to breathe; noisy breathing; use of accessory muscles to breathe; tripod position; abnormal breathing rate and rhythm; increased pulse rate; skin color changes; altered mental status. *(pp. 201-202)*
7. Carefully assess the patient's breathing to determine if it is adequate. Monitor it throughout the call. If you find respirations are inadequate, provide artificial ventilation immediately. Place the responsive patient with adequate breathing in a position of comfort. Administer oxygen, if you are trained and allowed to do so, by way of a nonrebreather mask at 12-15 liters per minute. Comfort and reassure the patient. If not done previously, activate the EMS system immediately. *(pp. 202-203)*
8. a *(p. 202)*
9. b, c *(pp. 203-204)*
10. d *(Chapter 9)*
11. d *(p. 201)*
12. Any five: When did the pain begin? Did anything cause or start the pain? What is the pain like? Where is the pain? Does the pain begin in one place and then seem to travel somewhere else? Where? Does anything relieve the pain? What? On a scale of 1-10, with 10 the worst, how bad is the pain? How long have you had the pain? *(p. 201)*
13. You should patch George into the defibrillator as soon as you determine that he is pulseless. Early defibrillation is one of the keys to surviving cardiac arrest. *(Chapter 7)*
14. George is in his 60s. According to his friends, he was playing golf when he clutched his chest and collapsed. I arrived to find George responsive but combative. His vital signs were respirations 32, pulse 32, BP 66/32, and skin pale, cool, and moist. As I was managing George, he lapsed into cardiac arrest. I immediately began CPR, and then delivered three shocks with the AED. He now has a carotid pulse, but he still requires ventilation. George's friends say he has a pacemaker and a history of heart problems. *(Chapter 9)*

Chapter 11: **Other Common Medical Complaints**

1. True *(p. 209)*
2. Every item in the list could be a cause of an altered mental status in a patient. *(p. 210)*
3. When you have determined the scene is safe, perform an initial assessment of the patient. If possible, administer high-flow oxygen. If necessary, help the patient get into a position of comfort. Attempt to gather an accurate patient history as soon as you can. Continue to monitor the patient's airway and breathing closely until the EMTs take over care. *(p. 210)*
4. A patient with an altered mental status may deteriorate rapidly. If you wait too long, the history—which could provide important clues to the cause of the patient's condition—could be lost to the EMTs and hospital staff who take over care. *(p. 210)*
5. Disagree. There are many reasons for altered mental status. One of the most common is decreased levels of oxygen in the patient's blood. So administering oxygen to this patient is a very good idea. All patients with altered mental status—even those suspected of having diabetes—should receive supplemental oxygen if possible. *(p. 210)*
6. altered mental status. *(p. 210)*
7. Any nine: sweet, fruity, or acetone-like breath; flushed, dry, warm skin or cool, clammy skin; hunger; thirst; rapid, weak pulse; altered mental status; staggering; slurred speech; frequent urination; headache; seizures; reports that patient has not taken prescribed diabetes medication. *(pp. 211-212)*
8. Medical identification tag, insulin in his or her refrigerator, presence of needles and syringes, presence of special needle containers. *(p. 213)*
9. Have you eaten today? Did you take your insulin? Have you been ill lately? Have you been particularly stressed lately? Are you having problems with any medication? *(p. 213)*
10. The four routes of exposure to poison are ingestion, inhalation, injection, and absorption. Examples of each may vary: ingestion—swallowing a handful of pills; inhalation—breathing in smoke from a fire; injection—sustaining a bite from a rattlesnake; absorption—rubbing against poison ivy leaves. *(pp. 214-217)*
11. Answers will vary: When did she eat the poison? How much did she eat? What exactly did she eat? Has she vomited? Have you given her anything to make her vomit? Have you given her any kind of antidote? *(p. 214)*
12. c *(p. 216)*
13. Disagree. All patients who have been exposed to carbon monoxide need medical care, even those who seem to have recovered. *(p. 216)*
14. The three types of signs or symptoms a patient who has had a stroke might exhibit are as follows (your examples may vary): inability to communicate—the patient may either fail to speak or fail to understand what is spoken; impairment in one part of the body—loss of muscle control on one side of the face or loss of movement on one entire side of the body; altered mental status—change in personality, seizures, unresponsiveness. *(p. 218)*
15. a. Agree
    b. Disagree. Stroke can affect any body system or any body part, including the respiratory system.
    c. Disagree. Generally, you should continue to talk to the patient even if he or she cannot speak. Stroke patients often can hear very well. So be reassuring, and explain to them what it is you are doing during emergency care. *(pp. 218-219)*
16. a, b, c. The first statement is careless and unprofessional. The second makes it seem that the level of care is dependent on the patient's performance, something the patient may not be able to control.

The third conveys a negative, pessimistic message. The fourth is reassuring and empathetic, and proposes a solution. *(pp. 218-219)*
17. **d** *(p. 219)*
18. **d** *(p. 220)*
19. 5, 1, 2, 3, 6, 4 *(pp. 221-222)*
20. Any six: abdominal pain, local or diffuse; colicky pain; abdominal tenderness, local or diffuse; anxiety; reluctance to move; loss of appetite; nausea, vomiting; fever; rigid, tense, or distended abdomen; signs of shock; vomiting blood, bright red or like coffee grounds; blood in the stool, bright red or tarry black. *(p. 222)*
21. This is called "guarding." This position helps to reduce tension on the muscles of the abdomen, which in turn helps to reduce pain. The patient may get in this position in response to abdominal pain. *(pp. 222-223)*
22. All except h are correct. *(p. 223)*
23. **b** *(p. 223)*
24. **d** *(p. 209)*
25. Any five (answers will vary): Can you tell me what day this is? The time of day? Where you are? What your name is? Do you have any pain? Do you remember collapsing? Do you feel any weakness or numbness? In your face? Arms? Legs? Are you having any vision problems? *(Chapter 9)*

Chapter 12: Environmental Emergencies

1. **a.** convection
   b. conduction
   c. radiation
   d. evaporation
   e. respiration *(pp. 229-230)*
2. 2, 3, 5, 4, 1 *(p. 232)*
3. False *(p. 230)*
4. Any five: Are there any signs of head or body trauma? Any allergies to medications? Is the patient taking any medication? Is there any possibility of alcohol or drug overdose? Is there any pertinent medical history? Any chronic medical problems that can be affected by the cold? When was the last time the patient ate or drank anything? Can the patient remember what she was doing prior to being found? How long was the patient out in the cold weather? *(Chapter 9)*
5. a, c, f *(pp. 231-232)*
6. Severely hypothermic patients are prone to ventricular fibrillation or sudden cardiac death when bounced or handled roughly. *(p. 231)*
7. **d.** The other signs are signs of a late or deep local cold injury. *(p. 232)*
8. **a** *(p. 233)*
9. Any five: muscle cramps; weakness, exhaustion; dizziness, faintness; rapid pulse rate that is strong at first, but becomes weak as damage progresses; headache; seizures; loss of appetite, nausea, vomiting; altered mental status, possibly unresponsiveness; skin may be moist, pale, and normal to cool or it may be hot and dry or hot and moist. *(pp. 234, 236)*
10. False. In heat stroke, a patient's skin is hot and dry or hot and moist. *(p. 236)*
11. Remove the patient from the hot environment. Administer oxygen if possible. Cool the patient by loosening or removing clothing and by fanning the surface of the body. Position the patient with legs elevated. Take vital signs frequently. *(p. 237)*
12. This firefighter may be in trouble. It is a hot day, and he has been fighting a major fire. He appears dazed and quite hot, and his response seems inappropriate given how uncomfortable he appears to be. Do not leave this patient. Insist that he allow you to examine him and treat him as necessary. Be gentle but persistent. *(pp. 234, 236)*
13. He may be suffering from heat stroke. *(pp. 234, 236)*
14. Disagree. Although this patient is probably dehydrated, he has been vomiting and has an altered mental status. If he should lapse into unresponsiveness and begin to vomit up the water you gave to him, the patient could experience a serious airway problem. Give him nothing by mouth. *(p. 237)*
15. Move the patient away from the hot environment. Perform an initial assessment and administer oxygen if possible. Place him in a supine position with legs elevated. While waiting for an ambulance to transport this patient to a hospital, cool him by removing clothing, applying cold packs to neck, armpits, and groin, sponging with water, and fanning aggressively. *(p. 237)*

Chapter 13: Psychological Emergencies and Crisis Intervention

1. **a.** Disagree. While this quote may show that the First Responder is trying to be empathetic and positive, he or she refers to the patient inappropriately as "pal" and "buddy," terms that may be perceived as condescending and phony. Call patients by their proper names.
   b. Disagree. This approach is threatening and berates the patient. No one wants to spend life in a wheelchair. While the First Responder says that he or she wants to help, the tone of this quote is anything but helpful. Calmly—and without threats—explain your reasons for wanting to take spinal precautions with a patient, as well as the potential risks of refusing this care. Ultimately, however, it is the patient's right to consent or withhold consent to your treatment.
   c. Agree. This is a good example of an approach that is calm, nonjudgmental, and straightforward. It informs the patient of what is happening and why.
   d. Agree. This approach is also nonjudgmental. The First Responder lets her know that he or she is there to help and that it is okay if Trish does not want to talk about the incident. The First Responder also keeps things simple. While it is clear that Trish does not want to describe the incident, the First Responder wisely moves to the simple question, "Were you hurt?"
   e. Disagree. This approach comes off sounding like a moralistic lecture. It is judgmental and chastises the patient for what is indeed inappropriate behavior. Avoid giving advice. *(pp. 245-247)*
2. **a, b.** Safety is always the top priority. Let law enforcement handle violent, weapon-wielding patients. Stay clear of the scene—and keep others

clear—until they have control of the patient.
(p. 245)

3. **d** *(p. 247)*
4. True *(p. 248)*
5. Any four: unresponsiveness, breathing difficulties or inability to maintain an open airway, abnormal or irregular pulse, fever, vomiting with an altered mental status or without a gag reflex, seizures. *(pp. 249-250)*
6. With a gloved hand, check the patient's mouth for partially dissolved pills or tablets. If you find any, remove them so they cannot block the patient's airway. Then smell the patient's breath for traces of alcohol. Ask the patient's friends or family what they know about the incident. Because signs and symptoms vary so widely and are so similar to many medical conditions, the most reliable indications of a drug- or alcohol-related emergency are likely to come from the scene and the patient history. *(pp. 250-251)*
7. Protect your own safety, maintain the patient's airway, and manage life-threatening conditions. *(p. 251)*
8. A few suggestions: "Hi, my name is ________ . I'm a First Responder with EMS, and I'm here to treat any injury you may have. After I help you, an ambulance will take you to the hospital. I want you to know that you are safe now. Do you hurt anywhere? I've been told that you were stabbed. Were you? Could I take a look at your stab wound?" *(pp. 252-253)*
9. You may want to talk with Rachel to calm her fears and better explain what the First Responder is doing. Given the physical, emotional, and psychological trauma she has experienced, she may be too disoriented to initially understand what the First Responder is trying to accomplish. Another strategy may be to find a female First Responder to manage Rachel's injuries. After being raped by a man, it may be too difficult for the patient to allow a male First Responder to touch her. *(pp. 252-253)*
10. Your treatment plan should include emergency care for the stab wound and treating any other injuries as necessary. Then you should support Rachel in whatever manner she needs until the ambulance arrives. Some sexual assault patients will want to talk. Others will want to remain silent. Gently gauge what Rachel appears to need in terms of emotional support. Do not be afraid to ask her, "How can I help you now, Rachel?" *(pp. 252-253)*

Chapter 14: **Bleeding and Shock**

1. **d** *(p. 259 and Chapter 2)*
2. Direct pressure, elevation, pressure points, splinting. *(p. 262)*
3. **a** *(p. 262)*
4. **c** *(pp. 263-264)*
5. **d** *(p. 265)*
6. Any five: discolored, tender, swollen, or hard tissue; increased respiratory and pulse rates; pale, cool, clammy skin; nausea and vomiting; vomitus with blood; thirst; changes in mental status; dark, tarry stools; tender, rigid, or distended abdomen; weakness, faintness, or dizziness. *(pp. 265-266)*
7. This patient probably died of internal injuries. Internal injuries can present with minor outward signs (in this case, minor abdominal pain). The picture becomes clear when you add up all of the elements of the call: his car was badly damaged, he complained of some abdominal pain, and his vital signs quickly deteriorated. *(pp. 265-266)*
8. **c, d** *(p. 267)*
9. **a, b, d** *(p. 267)*
10. **b, d** *(p. 268)*
11. **b** *(p. 268)*
12. **d** *(p. 267)*
13. To provide emergency care, take BSI precautions; maintain an open airway and adequate breathing; administer oxygen; prevent further blood loss; elevate the lower extremities if they are not injured; keep the patient warm; and do not give the patient anything to eat or drink. *(pp. 270-271)*
14. Make sure the scene is safe. *(Chapter 8)*
15. Assess the patient's ABCs, starting with her airway. Your next action will be to open her airway using a jaw-thrust maneuver. *(Chapter 5)*
16. Direct pressure, pressure point, and splinting. This injury is just below Paula's femoral pulse point. Applying direct pressure to the wound and to her femoral artery should control the bleeding. Elevating the area is really not practical as it is so close to the patient's pelvis. A tourniquet should only be used as a last resort and is rarely indicated. *(pp. 260, 262-264)*
17. Paula's most worrisome vital signs are her level of responsiveness and respiratory rate, which could indicate a severe head injury. The mechanism of injury suggests further internal injuries, and her skin condition indicates the possibility of shock. *(Chapter 9 and pp. 265-268)*
18. **a.** High
    b. High
    c. Low. Paula's medical history is much less important than managing her ABCs and major injuries.
    d. Low. Cuts and bruises can wait.
    e. High. Witnesses can provide important information about how Paula landed, whether or not she initially was conscious, had a seizure, etc.
    f. High. Always think safety.
    g. Low
    h. High
    i. Low
    j. High. The mechanisms of injury will help identify the patterns of injury to expect in Paula. *(Chapters 9 and 14)*

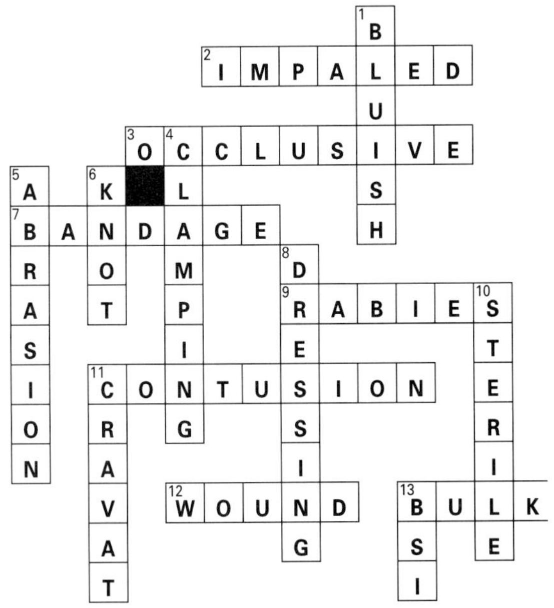

2. The patient's contusion would probably present as an area that is swollen and painful. It may exhibit ecchymosis (black and blue discoloration) and a hematoma (a lump with bluish discoloration). Cold compresses would help to relieve the pain and swelling. *(pp. 276-277)*

3. **a.** abrasion
   b. laceration
   c. puncture/penetration
   d. avulsion
   e. puncture/penetration (bite) or laceration (scratch)
   f. laceration
   g. laceration
   h. amputation
   i. puncture/penetration *(pp. 277-286)*

4. 5, 9, 8, 4, 3, 2, 6, 1, 7, 10 *(pp. 280, 285)*

5. Disagree. The location of the wound indicates possible injuries to the patient's lungs and major blood vessels. A two-inch (55 mm) blade is long enough to cause severe injuries. Wound severity should never be estimated by looking at external blood loss. Puncture wounds are rarely accompanied by significant external bleeding. Most bleeding will be internal. *(p. 280)*

6. **c.** Cutting an impaled object should only occur if it is an unmanageable size. *(p. 282)*

7. **d** *(p. 282)*

8. **a** *(p. 281)*

9. **a** *(p. 283)*

10. **c** *(p. 284)*

11. **a** *(p. 285)*

12. **d** *(p. 288)*

13. **b, d.** Bandages do not need to be sterile; they just need to be clean. *(p. 288)*

14. **a.** Disagree. If a patient tells you that the bandage is too tight, loosen it slightly. Chances are good that your bandaging job is cutting off circulation.
   b. Disagree. When bandaging wounds to a patient's arms or legs, always try to leave fingers and toes exposed so that you can assess circulation below the injury site.
   c. Agree. This First Responder is concerned about cutting off circulation to the patient's forearm and hand, but all important indicators—the patient's comfort level and distal color, temperature, and pulses—indicate that this is not the case.
   d. Agree. Wounds should be covered completely.
   e. Disagree. Triangular bandages do not make very good pressure bandages. They are not able to provide evenly distributed pressure to the wound, and often are too tight or too loose. A roller bandage—preferably the self-adhering type—would make a far superior pressure bandage. *(pp. 288-290)*

15. **c.** It can be very effective to focus a terrified patient on the tasks you are going to complete in order to help him or her. This statement also avoids judgments about the severity of the injury and whether or not the patient's response to being hurt is appropriate. *(p. 280)*

16. **d** *(p. 288)*

17. **c** *(pp. 288-290)*

18. Take BSI precautions! If you don't have a way to protect yourself, give bleeding control instructions to the child's mother. Do not risk contamination. *(Chapter 2)*

19. (Answers will vary.) Speak in a calm but firm voice. Use the child's name and focus him on quieting his screaming and thrashing about. Praise the child when he calms down and allows you to examine him. List the behaviors you need the child to exhibit so that you can help him. *(p. 280)*

20. Running water over the wound will only serve to keep the wound freely bleeding. It will not protect the patient from getting tetanus from the rusty pipe. The only real protection against tetanus is a vaccination.

21. The child has a three-inch (75 mm) laceration to his anterior thigh, beginning midway down his thigh and ending just proximal to his knee. The laceration is about one-inch (25 mm) deep. *(Chapter 4)*

22. Apply direct pressure and elevation. If the bleeding still does not stop, use a pressure point. *(Chapter 14)*

23. The patient is Danny Johnson. He is four years old. He lacerated his thigh on a rusty pipe while riding his bicycle. The laceration is about three-inches (75 mm) long and one-inch (25 mm) deep. It extends down his anterior thigh, beginning midway down the thigh and ending just proximal to his knee. When I arrived, the mother was irrigating the wound with a garden hose. The patient was quite agitated. I turned the water off, calmed the child, and controlled the bleeding using direct pressure and elevation. I estimate that the child has lost about 200 milliliters of blood. *(Chapter 9)*

Chapter 16: **Burn Emergencies**

1. Superficial burns: red skin and swelling
   Partial-thickness burns: red skin and blisters
   Full-thickness burns: charring, little or no pain
   (pp. 300, 302)

2. Using the "rule of nines," this patient has burned 22.5% of his body (anterior chest and abdomen, 18%; anterior arm, 4.5%). *(pp. 302, 303)*

3. **a.** Critical. Full-thickness burns involving the hands, feet, face, or genitals are considered critical. This patient's age also is a complicating factor.

   b. Minor. A superficial burn would be moderate only if it covered more than 50% of body surface area.

   c. Critical. Any burn complicated by a painful, swollen, deformed extremity is considered critical.

   d. Critical. The soot and cough suggest airway involvement. Any burn involving hands, feet, face, airway, or genitals in an infant or a child is considered critical.

   e. Minor. Even though this patient has a partial-thickness burn, it is isolated to a small portion of a non-critical area of his body.

   f. Minor. Although burns to the hands are often deemed critical, this is a minor burn to the back of the patient's hand and would not be considered critical. *(pp. 299, 300-303)*

4. **d** *(pp. 305, 307)*

5. 3, 6, 4, 1, 2, 7, 5 *(pp. 304-306)*

6. a, b, d, e, f, g, h, i, j *(p. 306)*

7. It is important to remove all items, such as the patient's rings and watch, that may retain heat or constrict a body part when the patient's burned skin swells. It also is important to remove any clothing near the burn sites. However, leave any clothing that is embedded in the burns. This clothing will have to be removed at the hospital by trained medical personnel. *(pp. 304-305)*

8. You are feeling the electrical field created by the power line. This is evidence that the line is still electrified and poses a serious hazard. Pull back until the power line is disabled. *(pp. 308-309)*

9. It is quite possible that this patient has breathing and circulation problems, spinal or other musculoskeletal injuries, external burns, and possibly internal injuries. You should have airway and breathing equipment, oxygen if possible, and burn dressings. *(pp. 308-309)*

10. Look for entry and exit wounds, in this case probably on the patient's arm or hand, leg or foot. (Imagine the farmer stepping down from the tractor, one hand on the tractor, one foot on the ground.) Cover the burns with dry, sterile dressings. *(pp. 308-309)*

11. The patient has severely compromised ABCs. His respiratory and pulse rates are too slow, and he has no measurable blood pressure. His airway should be opened with a jaw-thrust maneuver, and he needs to be ventilated with 100% oxygen immediately. In addition to his respiratory insufficiency, he appears to be in shock, so also keep him supine and warm. His burns and broken bones can be cared for when you get more help. *(pp. 304-306, 308-309)*

Chapter 17: **Musculoskeletal Injuries**

1. True *(p. 316)*

2. Any five: deformity or angulation; pain and tenderness; crepitus; swelling; bruising or discoloration; exposed bone ends; joint locked in position. *(pp. 316-317, 318)*

3. True *(p. 318)*

4. 5, 6, 1, 7, 3, 8, 2, 4 *(pp. 318-319)*

5. To prevent motion of bone fragments or dislocated joints; to minimize damage to surrounding tissues, nerves, blood vessels, and the injured bone itself; to help control bleeding and swelling; to help prevent shock; to reduce pain and suffering. *(p. 320)*

6. Disagree. You can't assess what you can't see. So cut away all clothing around the injury site before applying a splint. *(p. 321)*

7. The paragraph should read: If a long bone is injured, immobilize it and the joints above and below it. If a joint is injured, immobilize it and the bones above and below it. *(p. 321)*

8. Any three: compress nerves, tissues, and blood vessels under the splint; move displaced or broken bones; reduce blood flow below the injury site; delay transport. *(p. 321)*

9. STOP! Splint the injured arm in the position in which it was found. *(p. 321)*

10. Absolutely not. The elbow—and the knee—should be splinted in the position in which they are found. *(p. 323)*

11. **a.** *Patient A: #3.* He was wearing his seat belt. He has good vital signs, closed musculoskeletal injuries to one limb, and a small bump to his head. Perfusion in the injured extremities appears to be good. This patient should be treated last.

    b. *Patient B: #1.* He was not wearing a seat belt. This patient suffered a severe mechanism of injury. He is showing signs of shock and has an altered mental status. He has multiple extremity injuries, chest and pelvic injuries, and a large bruise to his head. He requires immediate transport.

    c. *Patient C: #2.* She was wearing a seat belt. She has good vital signs, but has suffered clavicle, wrist, and knee injuries. Of concern here is the lack of a pulse distal to her left knee injury. Perfusion appears to be good, except to her left foot. She needs immediate transport. *(Chapter 9)*

12. Agree. This EMT has recognized that Patient B is in shock and is suffering from severe injuries. This patient's broken humerus is the least of his problems. Critically injured trauma patients require immediate transport to a hospital if they are to survive. When managing this type of patient, strap painful, swollen, deformed injuries to the patient or to the long backboard. Remember, the patient's "Golden Hour" is ticking away. Prioritize. *(Chapter 14)*

13. Yes. Keep splinting as simple as possible. If she has immobilized the area herself (a "self-splint"), and your splinting efforts are causing her increasing pain, consider the splinting job done. *(p. 320)*

14. Splint the knee in the position found. Do not try to straighten it. *(pp. 326-327)*
15. Apply a pillow splint to the injured ankle after removing the patient's shoe and sock. *(pp. 327-328)*

Chapter 18: Injuries to the Head, Neck, and Spine

1. Any six: altered mental status; irregular breathing; open wounds to the scalp; penetrating wounds to the head; softness or depression of the skull; blood or cerebrospinal fluid leaking from ears or nose; facial bruises; bruising around the eyes or behind the ears; abnormal findings in pulse, movement, and sensation; headache severe enough to be disabling or which appears suddenly; nausea, vomiting; unequal pupil size with altered mental status; seizure activity. *(pp. 334-335)*
2. Disagree. Your job is not to diagnose a patient's injuries. Even if you were allowed to, there is no way to differentiate between a concussion and other head injuries in the field. While concussions are not life-threatening, many signs and symptoms of concussion are identical to the early signs and symptoms of serious brain injuries. *(pp. 334-337)*
3. a, b, c, d *(pp. 334-337)*
4. Any four: motor-vehicle collision; motorcycle crash; pedestrian-car crash; falls; diving accidents; hangings; blunt trauma; penetrating trauma to the head, neck, or torso; gunshot wounds; any speed sport accident, such as roller blading, bicycling, skiing, surfing, or sledding; any unresponsive trauma patient. *(p. 340)*
5. True *(p. 340)*
6. a *(p. 340)*
7. Any five: respiratory distress; tenderness at the site of injury on the spinal column; pain along the spinal column with movement; constant or intermittent pain without movement along the spinal column or in the lower legs; obvious deformity of the spine; soft-tissue injuries to the head, neck, shoulders, back, abdomen, or legs; numbness, weakness, or tingling in the arms or legs; loss of sensation or paralysis in the upper or lower extremities or below the injury site; incontinence; priapism. *(p. 340)*
8. True. So you must monitor the patient's airway and breathing continuously. *(p. 340)*
9. The paragraph should read: To manually stabilize a patient's cervical spine, you must place your gloved hands just behind the patient's ears. Then hold the patient's head firmly and steadily in a neutral, in-line position. *(p. 343)*
10. d *(p. 343)*
11. b *(p. 343)*
12. False. Stop at once if the responsive patient complains of pain or if you feel resistance in the unresponsive patient. Then stabilize the patient's head and neck in the position in which it was found. *(p. 343)*
13. False. Manual stabilization may be released when—and only when—the patient is completely immobilized from head to toe on a long backboard. *(p. 343)*

14. True. Cervical collars at best restrict movement by only 70%. The remaining 30% must be achieved by manual stabilization. *(p. 344)*
15. A cervical collar does not immobilize the patient. The First Responder should have maintained manual stabilization of the patient's head and neck until the patient was completely immobilized. Anything less constitutes inadequate care. *(pp. 343-345)*
16. Yes. When in doubt, take spinal precautions. That is, immediately stabilize the patient's head and neck. If you are allowed, apply a rigid cervical immobilization device and immobilize him on a long backboard. *(pp. 335, 340)*
17. 4, 5, 1, 12, 10, 11, 3, 9, 7, 6, 14, 8, 2, 13 *(pp. 340, 343, 345-347)*
18. False. Manual stabilization must be maintained until the patient is completely immobilized. The short backboard may be used to help immobilize a seated patient. It cannot replace immobilization on a long backboard. Complete immobilization on a long backboard is required to properly protect the patient's spine. *(pp. 345-347)*
19. Examples may include: when the scene is not safe, such as when there is threat of fire or explosion, a hostile crowd, extreme weather conditions; when life-saving care cannot be given because of the patient's location or position; when there is an inability to gain access to other patients who need life-saving care. *(pp. 348-349)*
20. a *(pp. 351-353)*
21. In general, a calm, direct approach is probably best. There are several onlookers who need to be calmed and directed—especially the one who is scaring your patient. It often helps to focus bystanders on a task, such as giving you the history of the event, fetching first aid materials, etc. You need to both establish control and calm people down so that you can properly care for the patient. *(Chapters 2, 8, and 9)*
22. First you need to stabilize John's head and neck. Then you need to perform an initial assessment. You will need an extra set of hands to accomplish all this. *(pp. 335, 340, and Chapter 9)*
23. d *(p. 340)*
24. Support John's airway, breathing, and circulation until the paramedics take over care. Be prepared to provide basic life support. *(p. 343)*
25. Disagree. Remember, John may have a spinal-cord injury. Moving him up to the roadway without the equipment necessary to properly immobilize him could further endanger John's life. It is certainly not worth the few minutes that may be saved by meeting the paramedics on the road rather than by the pool. Remember, even if John were to survive such a move, "quadriplegia is forever." *(p. 355)*
26. Your patient is a 16-year-old male named John. John dove into this pool and struck the top of his head on a rock outcropping. His friends pulled him from the water. I found him lying supine on the sand. He was awake but confused. I noted that he was breathing primarily from his diaphragm and that his pulse was 88. The only injury I found is a wound to the top of his head. Bleeding is controlled. I initially noted movement in his left arm only. Since my initial assessment and physical

exam, John's level of responsiveness has worsened. He is now unresponsive. His eyes have a pronounced gaze. His pulse has dropped to 44, and his breathing appears more labored. I am maintaining his head and neck in a neutral, in-line position. *(Chapter 9)*

Chapter 19: **Childbirth**

Crossword solution:

1. (across) U M B I L I C A L
3. (across) S A C ... 4. (across) S H O C K
6. (across) B I R T H
10. (across) U T E R U S
12. (across) P L A C E N T A S
14. (across) C R O W N I N G

2. (down) M E C O N I U M
5. (down) C E R V I X
7. (down) T O X E M I A
8. (down) P R O L A P S E D
9. (down) M U C O U S
11. (down) O B
13. (down) C O D

2. Place your gloved hand on the mother's abdomen, just above her navel. Feel the involuntary tightening and relaxing of the uterine muscles. Time these involuntary movements in seconds. Start from the moment the uterus first tightens until it is completely relaxed. Time the intervals in minutes from the start of one contraction to the start of the next. *(p. 362)*
3. **d** *(p. 362)*
4. Any five: Have you had a baby before? Are you having contractions? How far apart are they? Has the amniotic sac ruptured? If so, when? Do you feel the sensation of a bowel movement? Do you feel like the baby is ready to be born? *(p. 362)*
5. Any five: put on eyewear, a face mask, protective gloves, a disposable gown, and shoe coverings; handle soaked dressings, pads, and linens carefully, place them in separate bags that will not leak, and then seal and label the bags; scrub your arms, hands, and nails thoroughly before and after the delivery, even if you wore gloves. *(p. 363)*
6. **d** *(p. 364)*
7. Clean the area around the baby's mouth and nose once the head is delivered. Then clear the baby's airway by suctioning the mouth first and then the nose with a rubber suction syringe. Repeat if necessary. *(p. 364)*
8. False. Meconium staining can be life-threatening. If this occurs, you must consider requesting an advanced life-support team to assist. *(p. 364)*
9. **c** *(pp. 364-365)*
10. **a** *(p. 366)*
11. **a.** Rub the back gently or slap the soles of the feet. *(p. 366)*
12. **b** *(p. 366)*
13. **a** *(pp. 366-367)*
14. **a, b, c, d** *(p. 367)*

15. **c** *(p. 369)*
16. **c** *(pp. 369-370)*
17. It would probably be a good idea to see if one of the rescuers can move the station wagon to a safer location, preferably off the expressway. You need to work with the mother to calm her and reassure her and to help her focus on her labor. Her husband needs to be calmed and reassured as well. A rescuer should help him to support his wife by placing him by her head or somewhere else close to her. *(p. 363)*
18. Since this is her first baby and her contractions are still 6 minutes apart, there is probably time for transport to the hospital. *(p. 362)*
19. Recheck the contractions. See if they have changed in any way. If her contractions are 2 minutes apart or less and she feels the urge to push, birth may be imminent. Check to see if the baby's head is crowning at the vaginal opening. *(p. 362)*
20. The labor has progressed. The baby's head will appear at the opening of the birth canal very soon. *(p. 361)*
21. This baby needs to be ventilated. Provide the baby with small, controlled puffs to oxygenate her and to stimulate her to breathe. *(p. 366)*
22. Disagree. The mother and baby should be transported by an ambulance. Both patients need to be monitored closely until they reach the hospital. It is important for both to have their ABCs reassessed, especially the baby's. In addition, the mother still needs to pass the placenta. Caregivers will have more room to work in the ambulance, and it is better equipped should the mother or baby require any additional care.

Chapter 20: **Infants and Children**

1. The First Responder's approach is guaranteed to alienate and upset Katie's parents. He lacks any empathy for Katie's mother and does little to hide the fact that he sees her as a nuisance, a barrier to caring for Katie, rather than a resource. An appropriate response would be to empathize with Katie's mother. A seizure is scary to watch, especially when someone you love is convulsing in front of you. After reassuring her that the worst is probably over, focus on tapping Katie's mother for important patient history information. In addition, there is no one better qualified to calm Katie than her mother or father. Generally, allow parents to stay with their children. *(pp. 377-379)*
2. True *(p. 380)*
3. Any five: noisy breathing; cyanosis; flaring nostrils; retractions; use of accessory muscles to breathe; breathing with obvious effort; altered mental status. *(p. 380)*
4. **a** *(p. 380)*
5. **a.** Palpate the infant's brachial pulse.
   b. Palpate the unresponsive child's carotid or femoral pulse.
   c. Palpate the responsive child's radial or brachial pulse. *(p. 380)*
6. **b** *(p. 380)*

7. It is difficult to assess pain in infants and children. They may lack the body awareness and vocabulary necessary to describe it. Children also may not be able to separate the fear they feel from their physical condition. *(p. 381)*
8. **c** *(p. 382)*
9. **b.** When an infant's tongue relaxes, it can easily block the airway. Carefully position the airway in any infant with an altered mental status to avoid this problem. *(pp. 384-385)*
   c. Because of the larger head, the airway is more easily closed off when the patient is on his or her back. It may be necessary to place a thin pad under the shoulder in order to keep the patient's head in a neutral position and the airway open. Because of their larger heads, infants and children are more likely to suffer head and neck injuries, too. Always take spinal precautions for any infant or child who has suffered a mechanism of injury that suggests a possible head or spine injury. *(pp. 384-385)*
   d. Loss of even a small amount of blood may cause shock in an infant or a young child. Carefully monitor the vital signs of any infant or child patient who has experienced even slight external blood loss or who may have internal bleeding. *(pp. 384-385)*
   e. This makes pediatric patients more susceptible to hypothermia and dehydration, and more adversely affected by burns. Keep your pediatric patients warm. *(pp. 384-385)*
   f. Make sure that cervical collars fit correctly. Many children will not fit into even the shortest ones. Be prepared to use a rolled up towel in these cases. *(pp. 384-385)*
10. Any five: altered mental status; apathy, lack of vitality, inability to recognize a parent; delayed capillary refill; rapid or weak and thready pulse; pale, cool, clammy skin; rapid breathing; falling or low blood pressure (a late sign); absence of tears when crying. *(p. 387)*
11. **d** *(p. 390)*
12. True *(p. 390)*
13. Any six: When was the baby put in the crib? What was the last time the parents looked in on the baby? What was the position of the baby in the crib when found? What else was in the crib? Is there any medication present? What is the general health of the infant, recent illnesses, medications, or allergies? *(pp. 391-392)*
14. It is not appropriate. When at the scene of a suspected child abuse emergency, a First Responder should deal with the child's immediate medical emergency. This is not the time to be accusatory or confrontational. *(pp. 392-394)*
15. Lateesha's respirations, pulse, and blood pressure are all higher than normal. Normal ranges would be respirations 12-26, pulse 80-100, and blood pressure 96-98/70. *(p. 383)*
16. Any five: Is this the first time you have ever had trouble breathing? Is your breathing getting better? Is it getting worse? Do you have any pain in your body? In your chest? In your back? In your stomach? Do you take any medicine for your breathing? Do you take any other medicine? How is your

breathing right now? What were you doing when you began to have trouble breathing? *(Chapter 9)*
17. 7, 1, 6, 3, 4, 5, 8, 2. Note that the order of steps a (7), c (6), and g (8) may vary. *(Chapter 9)*

Chapter 21: **Lifting and Moving Patients**

1. Use your legs to lift, not your back. Keep the weight of the object as close to your body as possible. Align shoulders, hips, and feet. Reduce the height or distance you need to move the object. *(p. 400)*
2. **a** *(p. 400)*
3. **d** *(p. 402)*
4. **d** *(p. 402)*
5. **d** *(p. 402)*
6. An emergency move may be necessary if there is fire or threat of fire, explosion or threat of explosion, inability to protect the patient from other hazards at the scene, inability to gain access to other patients who need life-saving care, or inability to give life-saving care because of the patient's location or position. *(p. 403)*
7. True. *(p. 404)*
8. 5, 1, 3, 2, 4 *(p. 404)*
9. False. The extremity lift should be used only when the patient has no injuries to his arms or legs. *(p. 405)*
10. **a, c** *(p. 410)*
11. **a** *(p. 411)*
12. **a** *(p. 412)*
13. Among your responsibilities are to guard your personal health and safety, to maintain a caring attitude, and to maintain your own composure. *(Chapters 1, 2, and 9)*
14. You would need to consider if there is an immediate danger to the patient. In this case, a determining factor may be whether or not the structure is stable. *(pp. 403-404)*
15. **a.** No. There does not appear to be a threat to life.
    b. Yes, you probably should move patient #2 and patient #3 in order to gain access to patient #4. Patient #4 may need to be moved in order to provide life-saving emergency care. If he needs artificial ventilation or CPR, you may have to move him into the correct position.
    c. No, because there appears to be no immediate threat to life. *(pp. 403-404)*

Chapter 22: **Multlple-Casualty Incidents and Incident Management**

1. Command—responsible for direction and oversight of all incident activities; operations—responsible for carrying out the goals of the mission as set by Command; planning—responsible for gathering and evaluating information about the incident, including the status of rescuers; logistics—responsible for providing facilities, services, and materials to support response at an emergency scene; finance/administration—responsible for costs and financial aspects of an incident. *(pp. 420-421)*
2. **b** *(p. 422)*

3. Number of patients, including the "walking wounded"; scene hazards; apparent patient priorities; need for extrication; number of ambulances required; other factors affecting the scene and resources needed to address them; areas to stage resources. *(p. 423)*

4. **a.** Priority 1
   b. Priority 3
   c. Priority 2
   d. Priority 2
   e. Priority 1
   f. Priority 3
   g. Priority 1
   h. Priority 1
   i. Priority 3
   j. Priority 1
   k. Priority 3
   l. Priority 1
   m. Priority 4 *(p. 427)*

5. Patient 1: d
   Patient 2: d
   Patient 3: a

6. What are the scene hazards? How many patients are there? What priority are these patients? What type of extrication effort do they need? How many ambulances are needed? Where should the incoming resources be staged? Are there any other factors affecting the scene? Are there any other resources needed to manage the incident? *(p. 423)*

7. Patient a: Priority 1
   Patient b: Priority 1
   Patient c: Priority 2
   Patient d: Priority 4
   Patient e: Priority 1
   Patient f: Priority 4
   Patient g: Priority 2

8. At least four ambulances are needed. Each of the priority-1 patients needs an ambulance. The two priority-2 patients may be transported together, however, because both of these patients could develop breathing problems very quickly. Five ambulances would be better.

Chapter 23: EMS Operations

1. **b** *(p. 437)*
2. **f** *(p. 438)*
3. **a, d, e** *(p. 438)*
4. Any four: know all local and state guidelines related to driving emergency vehicles; when possible, travel in pairs; when backing up, do so slowly and carefully, use all available mirrors, and have your partner take a position in the rear to act as spotter; know the territory and take alternative routes to avoid potential problems; exercise extra caution when traveling in traffic; plan for stopping distance; avoid sudden braking at high speeds; practice special caution on curves and hills. *(pp. 439–440)*
5. False. Too many emergency responders are injured because they have done this. Keep your seat belt on until the vehicle has come to a full stop. *(p. 440)*
6. True *(p. 440)*

7. Keep the windows closed while the siren is on; wear ear plugs or ear muffs; move the siren speakers from the top of the cab to the front grille. *(p. 440)*
8. False *(p. 441)*
9. He should put on an impact-resistant protective helmet with reflective tape and a strap under the chin. *(p. 442)*
10. Any five: know the location; plan a route; wear seat belts; exercise due regard for safety of others; use lights and siren; use a spotter to back up the vehicle; avoid excessive speed; park on the shoulder or in a driveway. *(pp. 439–443)*
11. To channel traffic around the scene to avoid additional collisions; to minimize disruption of traffic flow when possible; to clear the scene for safe arrival of additional emergency vehicles. *(p. 442)*
12. Have all responders wear reflective equipment; place the cones or flares 10–15 feet (3–5 m) apart and approximately 100 feet (30 m) into traffic; place them at the beginning of a curve or the crest of a hill. *(p. 442)*

Chapter 24: Hazardous Materials

1. Identify the emergency as a hazmat incident; identify the hazardous materials; establish command and control zones; establish a medical treatment sector. *(p. 453)*
2. **a.** The first step is always to take a position from a safe distance and then assess the situation. If you do this prior to contacting EMS, you will have more information to give them regarding the specific nature and circumstances of the incident. *(pp. 453–455)*
3. Any three: smoking or self-igniting materials; extraordinary fire conditions; boiling or spattering of materials that have not been heated; wavy or unusual vapors over a container of liquid material; colored vapor clouds; frost near a container leak; unusual condition of containers. *(p. 454)*
4. **c** *(p. 454)*
5. **a** *(p. 454)*
6. The nature and exact location of the incident; a description of the incident, including any potential for fire or explosion; the number of patients involved; a request for additional help, such as fire, police, EMS, and hazmat support; suggestion for the way rescuers can approach the scene; if possible, identify the hazardous materials and the severity of the situation. *(p. 454)*
7. **b** *(p. 455)*
8. **c** *(p. 455)*
9. You can alert the responding hazmat team as to the type of substance leaking from the truck and the approximate area of contamination. You can deny entry to the scene and possibly set up a medical treatment sector. However, you should not enter the scene to render aid to the driver or other injured people because you lack the equipment and training to do so. While it is difficult to stand by while an injured patient is unattended, you must not risk exposure to the acid. *(pp. 453–458)*
10. **b** *(pp. 453–454)*

11. Never deviate from your EMS system's hazmat response plan. Never discontinue it based on partial or sketchy information. Cutting corners in an emergency response to a hazardous material can lead to lost lives and bungled operations. Stick to the plan no matter what the material turns out to be.
12. Deny them access. A search of the shed requires rescuers equipped with self-contained breathing apparatus and specialized training. Your job is to protect those who have escaped. *(pp. 453-455, 458)*

Chapter 25: **Fireground Rehabllitation**

1. True *(p. 464)*
2. A fatigued firefighter places himself and other firefighters in that crew at risk, so the company officer's decision to send Bill to rehab was correct. However, the entire crew should report to rehab because if one member is at his limits of endurance, then others in that same crew may be, too. *(pp. 467-468)*
3. **b, c, d.** Item "a" is incorrect because you should be "upwind of the hot zone," not downwind; you don't want smoke and other hazardous materials to endanger rescuers. Item "e" is incorrect because you want to have the staging area close enough for easy access in case ambulance transport is needed. *(p. 466)*
4. **d** *(p. 468)*
5. False. There should be a single entry/exit point in order to track rescuers accurately. *(p. 467)*
6. **a** *(p. 468)*
7. **b** *(pp. 468-469)*
8. Identify rescuers entering rehab who are at risk for stress- and heat-related illness; medically monitor rescuers and determine if they are fit to return to active duty, require more hydration and rest, or require transport for further evaluation and treatment; assure accountability; update the safety officer or incident commander on the status of rehab. *(pp. 465-466)*
9. When any rescuer feels as if he has reached his limit (then all of his crew members should report, too); after going through two 30-minute SCBA air cylinders; after 45 minutes of active fire suppression duty. *(pp. 467-468)*
10. Any eight: chest pain; shortness of breath; altered mental status; skin that is hot and either dry or moist; oral temperature greater than 101°F (38.3°C); irregular pulse; pulse greater than 150 at any time; pulse greater than 140 after cool-down; systolic BP greater than 200 mm Hg after cool-down; diastolic BP greater than 130 mm Hg at any time. *(p. 470)*

Chapter 26: **EMS Rescue Operations**

1. Since you are alone, you will not be able to extricate the patient. Make sure the scene is safe. Set out flares to warn oncoming motorists. Make sure that the car's ignition is turned off and that there is no threat of fire. Make sure that the vehicle is stabilized. If possible, gain access to the patient and assess his ABCs. Support his ABCs, if necessary, and apply oxygen if it is available. Attempt to keep his head and neck in a neutral position. *(pp. 477-482)*
2. **a, b, c, e.** Item "d" is not true; you should position flares in both directions. *(p. 478)*
3. False. *(pp. 479-480)*
4. **b, c.** Even if the proper equipment were immediately available, removing the windshield or cutting off the roof of the car will take too much time, given the appearance of the patient. *(p. 480)*
5. True *(p. 480)*
6. Drownings that occur in cold water have resulted in successful resuscitations, even up to an hour after submersion. *(p. 483)*
7. You are a good swimmer; you are specially trained in water rescue; you are wearing a personal flotation device; you are accompanied by other rescuers. *(p. 483)*
8. *Throw*—Throw an object that floats. If possible, tie a rope to it, toss it to the patient, and pull on the rope to tow the patient in. *Row*—If the patient is too far to reach from shore, then use a boat to get closer to the patient. *Go*—If reaching, throwing, and rowing are not possible, then swim to the patient. *(p. 483)*
9. Establish who will be responsible for functions such as assessing the patient, ventilating the patient, gathering a patient history, and so on. You can also review your game plan for controlling the scene and interfacing with the other responding agencies. *(Chapter 8)*
10. Any three: reposition her head and open her airway using a jaw-thrust maneuver; reinsert the oropharyngeal airway after checking that it is the correct size; evaluate the patient for a foreign body airway obstruction; check that your ventilation equipment is not faulty (holes in the BVM, etc.); check that the BVM fits her face correctly. If after all of the above, consider using a head-tilt/chin-lift maneuver to better open her airway. While it is important that you protect her spine, it is more important that you ventilate her enough to keep her alive. *(Chapter 5)*
11. It is important that you be honest with the parent about the condition of his or her child. It is also important that you reassure the parent that you are doing everything you can to help. In this instance you may want to say the following: "Your daughter's heart is beating, but she is not breathing, so we are concentrating on breathing for her, using 100% oxygen. We are also suctioning her mouth to keep it free of water and food from her stomach. We are holding her neck and back to protect them from any possible injuries. She isn't awake right now, but we are doing everything we can to help maintain her breathing and heartbeat. The paramedics will be here any minute, and they will be transporting her to the closest hospital." Do not pronounce any judgments about the child's final outcome. It is best not to hypothesize about whether or not the child will survive. Leave this up to the medical team at the hospital. *(Chapter 20)*
12. 5, 3, 1, 2, 4, 6, 7 *(Chapter 9)*